The Public Health Approach

The Public Health Approach

Population Thinking from the Black Death to COVID-19

Alfredo Morabia, MD

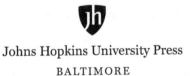

Johns Hopkins University Press

BALTIMORE

Johns Hopkins University Press
2715 North Charles Street
Baltimore, Maryland 21218
www.press.jhu.edu

Library of Congress Cataloging-in-Publication Data

Names: Morabia, Alfredo, author.
Title: The public health approach : population thinking from
   the Black Death to COVID-19 / Alfredo Morabia.
Description: Baltimore : Johns Hopkins University Press, 2023. |
   Includes bibliographical references and index.
Identifiers: LCCN 2022042962 | ISBN 9781421446783
   (paperback ; alk. paper) | ISBN 9781421446790 (ebook)
Subjects: MESH: Public Health Practice—history | Communicable
   Disease Control—history | Population Health—history |
   Epidemiologic Methods | Social Determinants of Health—history
Classification: LCC RA418 | NLM WA 11.1 | DDC 362.1—dc23/
   eng/20230405
LC record available at https://lccn.loc.gov/2022042962

A catalog record for this book is available from the British Library.

*Special discounts are available for bulk purchases of this book. For more
information, please contact Special Sales at specialsales@jh.edu.*

To Linda,
With love

Contents

Figures

The Public Health Approach

Prologue

There is much to criticize in the response to the COVID-19 pandemic in the United States. Many more lives could have been saved, and the United States ranks worse than other wealthy countries in terms of mortality and vaccination rates. The pandemic intensified health inequities that were already deeper in the United States than in any other wealthy country. But these insufficient aspects of the response should not overshadow the remarkable achievements of public health officials and scientists in multiple disciplines: they devised and implemented a safe prevention strategy that reached hundreds of millions of people.

The COVID-19 vaccination campaign in the United States and many other countries has been a success of historical dimensions. In the first three months of 2021, about 200 million Americans were vaccinated at least once. As of September 22, 2022, 84% of Americans age 5 years and up had received at least one dose of the vaccine and 72% had had two doses, which is considered fully vaccinated. More than 95% of people age 65 and up had received at least one dose, and about 92% of that group were fully vaccinated.[1] Harmful effects of the COVID-19 vaccines have been rare. According to one study, "Safety data from more than 298 million doses of mRNA COVID-19 vaccine administered in the first 6 months of the US vaccination program show that most reported adverse events were mild and short in duration."[2] Risks of anaphylaxis, thrombosis with thrombocytopenia syndrome, Guillain-Barré syndrome, and death after vaccination were extremely rare.[3] During the wave of the pandemic following the introduction of the vaccine, the Texas Department of State Health Services reported that vaccinated persons were 20 times less likely to succumb to an infection than unvaccinated people were.[4] There has rarely been as much evidence for the safety and effectiveness of any vaccine, drug, or treatment.

A vigorous vaccination campaign involving public health officials from the local to the federal level overcame many hurdles to reach people who wanted to be vaccinated. Not only have millions of hospitalizations and deaths been prevented,[5] but the knowledge public health professionals gained as a result of combining logistics and communication has the potential to strengthen processes for controlling other epidemics such as opioid use, obesity, smoking, diabetes, and HIV/AIDS. In the COVID-19 pandemic response, public health rose to the challenges.

Yet even when people trust the recommendations of public health officials and, for example, agree to have their children vaccinated against childhood diseases or to get vaccinated against COVID-19 themselves, the methods that underlie such a safe collective response to a collective threat remain mysterious to most members of the general public. There is a simple, fundamental reason for that. Public health officials are population thinkers—they draw a type of knowledge from the study of populations that enables them to achieve such feats. This knowledge is not something most people are familiar with. Most people extrapolate knowledge from their personal experiences and rarely consider the population dimension of health.

This book is about how public health professionals think. It begins by explaining what public health is and why its focus on populations differs from the focus of medicine on individuals. There is no clear evidence that the population dimension of health was known before the seventeenth century, when it was first described. Step-by-step, a new strategy for understanding and effectively controlling epidemics of disease emerged that I refer to as the Public Health Approach. The chapters of this book describe how its principles were discovered and then improved by trial and error during epidemics of bubonic plague in the seventeenth century, smallpox in the eighteenth century, cholera in the nineteenth century, tuberculosis and HIV/AIDS in the twentieth century, and the SARS-CoV-2 pandemic of the twenty-first century. Other chapters describe how the Public Health Approach was eventually used to address behavioral (e.g., smoking tobacco) and social (e.g., unemployment, police brutality) determinants of health.

Population Thinking

Without specific training, most people think in individual terms. For example, someone may mistakenly believe that cigarettes cannot cause lung cancer because a neighbor who is 80 still smokes and has not developed cancer or that the COVID-19 vaccine kills because someone they know died 24 hours after receiving a first vaccine shot. However, observing one person is not very informative for another person because everyone has unique biological characteristics that have been exposed to a specific set of social and environmental factors.

The problem with individual-level thinking is that it extrapolates from anecdotes, which are unsystematic observations, and ignores what is happening for the whole population. An 80-year-old smoker cannot be representative of all smokers for many reasons. Here is just one: natural selection and DNA recombination may have resulted in that individual reacting differently to the carcinogens contained in the smoke of tobacco than smokers who die at a younger age. To know whether cigarettes cause lung cancer, one must compare the occurrence of lung cancer in smokers and non-smokers. In contrast to the future health of individuals, the future health of groups of people is predictable. If two groups of people are carefully selected to be comparable on average in terms of key factors such as age and gender, they may be expected to have—on average—the same risk of lung cancer prior to being exposed—or not exposed—to tobacco carcinogens. Every comparative study has found that smokers are much more likely than nonsmokers to get lung cancer. We can say that cigarette smoking causes lung cancer because smokers taken as a group are more likely to develop lung cancer (say, 10% of them over their lifetime) than nonsmokers, of whom only 0.5% develop lung cancer.

For the same reason, when millions of persons are vaccinated, some deaths may occur by chance in the days following the injection. The tragic death of baseball player Hank Aaron is a case in point. He received a COVID-19 vaccination at age 86. Two weeks later, he died from a massive stroke. Several medical experts agreed that Aaron's vaccination had nothing to do with his stroke.[6] Comparing the mortality rate of vaccinated with nonvaccinated people at age 86 revealed whether Aaron's term death was within expectation regardless of whether or not he received the vaccine. As Michael Osterholm, epidemiologist and director of the Center for Infectious Disease Research and Policy at the University of Minnesota, explained, "If you look at heart attacks in the United States and you look at the incidence per 10 million people getting vaccinated . . . which is roughly the number we have vaccinated in the U. S., in that age group from 55 to 64, you would expect to see 793 individuals die from a heart attack in that week following vaccination, just by chance alone, if vaccination never occurred."[7] This reasoning is called population thinking.

Observing aggregated individuals is informative because a group has properties that its individual members do not have. When a population is enumerated, it becomes a statistical entity.

Its progression, spontaneously or in response to preventive measures and treatments, appears to be subject to some rules. That predictable progression confers the type of regularity needed for scientific comparisons. Populations can be compared, and these comparisons open up a vast domain of scientific knowledge that can provide answers to questions such as What is causing an epidemic? Who is most affected? Is this mode of prevention, control, or treatment effective? and How frequent are the side effects of treatments? The knowledge public health professionals use derives from the study, analysis, and comparison of populations. Looking beyond individuals enables public health professionals to build effective and safe strategies for controlling a threat to our collective health.

The gateway to the Public Health Approach is a switch from thinking about individuals to thinking about populations when responding to a question about health. These two forms of thinking sometimes clash. Individual thinking can lead to conclusions (e.g., "tobacco does not cause lung cancer," or "vaccines kill") that are not accurate when the lens shifts to a population perspective.

The tension between individual and population thinking is not specific to public health. In his book *Outliers: The Story of Success*, Malcolm Gladwell "look[ed] *beyond* the individual" (his emphasis)[8] to explain some successes. For example, he looked at the trajectory of individual Canadian hockey players who appeared to have been selected because they were the most gifted for the game in their age cohort. However, when he looked at the players of Canadian junior hockey leagues as a group, he noticed that most were born in the months of January through April. This clustering of birth months may be related to the fact that children in Canada begin to play hockey as soon as they reach age 5 after January 1. At this young age, those born in January are likely to be stronger, taller, and so on, than those born in December of the same year. The biological advantage of the few months' difference is increased when the oldest members of age cohorts are selected for hockey teams. *Outliers* switches from individual to population thinking to reveal patterns that can only be seen "beyond the individual." Gladwell's use of population thinking about hockey players included the comparative step: he suggested that on teams that do not begin their selection process on January 1 of the year the child reaches age 5, the birth-dates of the players are more evenly distributed across the twelve months.

The first time a human being had access to population patterns that were invisible at the individual level took place 360 years ago. This leap from an individual to a population form of logic was explicitly described in a 1662 publication that showed that, unexpectedly, deaths from some causes occurred with a predictable frequency across time in the City of London.[9] The tabulation of the series of mortality data for an entire population over decades revealed that about 20% of the deaths in the population of London were annually due to "consumption and cough," mostly from tuberculosis. This regularity was surprising. Illness and death had until then always seemed to be unpredictable. Yet looking at the whole of London indicated that the annual numbers of deaths for a given year were informative about the annual number of deaths from tuberculosis for the following year. The future health of Londoners was predictable. That phenomenon was impossible to explain except for the fact that the entire population of London, collectively, had unique properties that each Londoner did not individually have.

Before 1662, the common belief of human civilizations was that deaths from disease occurred by chance or by providential or divine intervention. Deaths were commonly referred to as "casualties"—that is, events occurring unpredictably. In antiquity, physicians established only the obvious links between specific exposures and symptoms. For instance, it was common knowledge that people living in marshland areas suffered from periodic fevers, which we know today are caused by a disease called malaria. Most illnesses, however, seemed to result from a complex mix of environmental and individual factors that made their occurrence unpredictable. Governments in antiquity and the Middle Ages could expect that providing clean water, sewers, and public baths would have beneficial impacts on individual well-being, but they could not link clean water, sewers, and public baths to specific diseases. The analysis of the London data was a game changer: a comparison of erratic occurrences of the plague to the regular occurrence of tuberculosis pointed toward different causes and modes of transmission for these two diseases and therefore toward different interventions to control them. The same tools are used now to assess the efficacy of personal protective equipment, establish the safety of some vaccines against COVID-19, and deploy mass strategies for disease prevention.

Becoming a Population Thinker

Three reasons explain why population thinking yields new knowledge that is not available to individual thinking. The first is that regularities stem from the aggregate effect of causes acting differently on individuals who are intrinsically unique. Although gender, residence, class, time, and genetic background act on individuals in unique ways, they have health effects that are shared by multiple individuals. These effects can stand out beyond residual individual differences when an entire group is studied.

Second, the results of population thinking can be explained by the theory of probability, which dates to the work in the seventeenth century of philosopher Blaise Pascal (1623–1662) and scientist Christiaan Huygens (1629–1695). The technical explanation is encapsulated in the notion of risk. Statistically, a risk is a measure of the frequency of a health event or, as Virginia Berridge and co-authors nicely put it, the frequency of "a future harm that can be avoided or mitigated"[10] The term "risk" may be used more commonly than "probability," but they mean the same thing. For example, say the risk of succumbing from COVID-19 among unvaccinated people infected by SARS-CoV-2 in 2020 was 1%, that is, one death for every 100 people infected. A 1% risk allows for an accurate prediction at the population level. Policymakers can use it to plan for the hospital infrastructure that will be needed to take care of the sick. Yet it is impossible to predict which individuals will be the next COVID-19 victims. Risks can also be compared and can yield clues about causal connections. When, as already mentioned, the Texas Department of State Health Services stated that "Texas data shows unvaccinated people are 20 times more likely to die from COVID-19," it was indicating what the ratio of risks for unvaccinated people was to the risks for vaccinated people.[11]

Finally, a metaphor may provide an intuitive explanation for why population thinking leads to new insights. Imagine populations as "superindividuals" that include many individuals yet have properties that each individual does not have. Individuals commonly talk about "their" risk of getting sick, but there is no such thing as an "individual" risk. An individual cannot predict whether they will be the 1 who will die from COVID-19 if infected or among the 99 who won't. In contrast, as a group or superindividual, a collective of infected individuals have an objective risk of succumbing to COVID-19: 1 will die for every 99 who will survive. Chapter 3 shows that this was the vision John Graunt had when he pioneered the analysis of mortality data in 1662. The City of London appeared to him as a superindividual. He considered the "fitness for long life" of the superindividual that was the population of London and "the wholesomeness of its food."[12] Chapter 8 shows that the same metaphor was implied in the mass prevention strategy epidemiologist Geoffrey Rose (1926–1993) promoted. Rose argued that extreme health behaviors, for instance, heavy smoking or heavy drinking, were more common or less common according to how much the whole community typically smoked or drank. As a result, the whole community, as a superindividual, had to rally to modify its behaviors if it wanted to reduce the fraction of its people who drank excessively, for example. Policies that aimed to reduce smoking or consumption of alcohol had to target everyone in order to reduce the frequency of extreme behaviors. Such a goal can be reached by regulating the availability, quality (e.g., alcohol or carcinogens content), and/or price of alcohol and tobacco. If nonsmoking becomes 'normal', then it is much less necessary to keep on persuading individuals to stop smoking or not to start the habit.[13] This mass strategy differs from a strategy that focuses only on the individuals of the subgroup of the population that is exhibiting extreme behaviors. That approach would be more logical in medicine: physicians preferentially treat individuals at high risk of disease or of death. In his groundbreaking book *The Strategy of Preventive Medicine*, Geoffrey Rose translated a quotation from Fyodor Dostoevsky's *The Brothers Karamazov* in an epigraph that is a great fit for the Public Health Approach: "we are all responsible to all for all."[14]

The mental switch from individual thinking to population thinking was indispensable for the emergence of a modern public health strategy that seeks to protect the health of all, but it was not sufficient. Its application was tested and challenged over the centuries. In each historical case this book examines, the people who switched their perspective and understood the Public Health Approach did not have specific religious or political traits. Consider Boston in 1721, when a catastrophic epidemic of smallpox hit the city. It was the clergy who urged doctors to immunize everyone using variolation, the ancestor of vaccines. Medical doctors were opposed to this strategy. Similarly, in the United Kingdom and the United States in the nineteenth century, certain public health reformers were opposed to quarantines, lockdowns, and shutting down the economy during pandemics of cholera, while laboratory scientists promoted these strategies. Agreeing to address the COVID-19 epidemic collectively by wearing masks, practicing physical distancing, washing hands, and later getting vaccinated goes beyond political and religious beliefs.

The history of the Public Health Approach suggests that an understanding of how public health professionals think may be the key to successful collective public health interventions. People are more likely to consider public health recommendations if they understand their underlying rationale. The COVID-19 pandemic has generated a universal discussion about the relevance of public health that has created favorable terrain for explaining the principles of the Public Health Approach to everyone. That is what this book is about.

Chapter 1

Public Health

What is public health? The question is less naïve than it seems. Ask people around you. I often get surprising answers, the most common one being that it is health care for the poor—that is, the care one gets when one cannot afford "private health." The public is familiar with vaccines, clean air, clean water, control of toxic waste, or controlling youth access to tobacco, but many do not see these goals as necessarily linked to public health. This is not new. Twenty-five years ago, Barry Levy, a former president of the American Public Health Association, aptly concluded from a 1996 Harris Poll that more Americans were familiar with the goals of public health and supported those goals than could recognize the term "public health."[1] A poll conducted in 2021 on the same topic generated similar answers but also revealed wide differences within the population.[2] Blacks and Latinos considered housing, homelessness, racism, and gun violence to be main responsibilities for public health agencies much more frequently than non-Hispanic whites did. John Kasich, former governor of Ohio, observed that public health officials do their work so modestly that until there is a disaster, people don't realize how much behind-the-scenes preventive work is done to protect them.[3] This is a concerning disconnect.

Policymakers and health practitioners use the term "public health" every day, but their constituencies may not understand exactly what they are talking about. A definition of public health is therefore warranted.

Public health has two main characteristics: a focus on the health of populations and government enforcement of public health policies and mandates. In contrast, medicine focuses on the health of individual patients, and the advice that doctors give their patients cannot be enforced. Still, too many people equate public health prescriptions, such as a vaccine mandate, with a doctor's prescription. They believe incorrectly that the same medical freedom applies to both when it does not.

Public Health and the Health of Populations

Public health uses a population lens to protect the health of individuals from collective threats that an individual cannot control. Since surveys suggest that it is often understood as government-funded *health care* for the poor who cannot afford to pay for health insurance, let's start by stressing that public health is *not* the opposite of private health. The expression "public health" itself may be faulty, because it creates a false dichotomy, public versus private health, instead of an apt one, population health versus individual health.[4]

The widespread belief that public health is health care for the poor has some rational and historical bases. Social inequities are a major cause of ill-health, disease, and shorter lives. Ensuring that disadvantaged populations have access to resources that affect their health is within the scope of this definition. When governments in antiquity or the Middle Ages were funding public doctors, they were providing access to health care for the poor. In the United States, Medicaid; the Special Supplemental Nutrition Program for Women, Infants, and Children (WIC); the Supplemental Nutrition Assistance Program (SNAP); and community health centers are contemporary components of public health. They primarily benefit the disadvantaged by providing access to health care, food, housing, and other essentials. People who are economically better off have other ways, and indeed often private ways, to satisfy their needs thanks to their income or the private insurance they can afford or that their employers provide. In all these examples, public health programs reduce inequities in access to services.

Public health is different from the individualized care doctors have been providing to sick patients for at least 4,000 years. When a doctor investigates the complaints of a patient and eventually proposes a treatment, that is individual health care, not public health. The patient can choose to accept or refuse the proposed treatment. That is their private, individual decision. That is medical freedom. When society or government institutions establish legal and ethical rules to control an epidemic; to provide access to vaccines, clean air, and clean water; to control how toxic waste is handled; or to inform the public about the health risks of consuming alcohol and tobacco and the protective effects of physical activity, that is public health. A collective threat has been identified that requires a collective response: everyone in the community must be able to benefit from that response or be required to comply with it. Individuals are powerless against these threats.

Public health covers an extremely vast domain. COVID-19 brought public health to the daily scrutiny of many more people than was the case before 2020. The pandemic illustrated how public health scientists assess risks of infections and deaths, estimate time for symptoms to develop, assess whether a treatment or personal protective equipment will work, and determine the effectiveness of vaccination campaigns. Before SARS-CoV-2, the history of public health overlapped with that of many epidemics such as measles, whooping cough, poliomyelitis, tetanus, cholera, tuberculosis, typhoid, typhus, and HIV/AIDS, among many other diseases. However, public health does not only deal with epidemics of infectious diseases. Scientists and officials also deal with epidemics of unhealthy behaviors, such as the use of tobacco, which shortens the lives of smokers due to cancer and respiratory and cardiovascular diseases. Tobacco smoking has been substantially reduced in many societies, even though it was a ubiquitous behavior in the 1950s. Public health deals with environmental exposures that can be prevented, for example, by enforcing clean air, clean water, removal of sewage, and decent housing. More recently, public health scientists have been exploring ways to mitigate the effects of social determinants of health, such as racism and capitalism. What all these public health interventions have in common is an ability to identify problems and solve them at the level of populations because they cannot be solved at the level of individuals.

Public Health Involves
Government Interventions

The second important feature of public health is that it can have the force of law through legislation, regulation, or public health orders. As Mark Rothstein has noted, "The key element of public health is the role of the government—its power and obligation to invoke mandatory or coercive measures to eliminate a threat to the public's health."[5] This form of regulation goes back to fifteenth-century Italy and was formalized in the late eighteenth century.[6] In his groundbreaking volume, *A System of a Complete Health Policy*,[7] Johann Peter Frank (1745–1821), a German physician, hygienist, and teacher, recommended that governments introduce laws regulating parenthood, the manual labor of women, children's education, and hygiene in schools. The goal of these recommendations was to alleviate the extreme misery of large segments of populations.

Laws and actions and their beneficial consequences are the hallmarks of public health. In the nineteenth century, sanitary reformers in Britain and the United States sought public interventions such as building sewers and removing garbage to eliminate the sources of stench in the air, which they believed caused sickness and death in the poor neighborhoods of the cities. The qualifier "sanitary," from the Latin *sanitas*, which means health, became associated with many government activities that were directly relevant to health, such as sanitary laws and sanitary inspections. Toilets became known as sanitary installations. By eliminating the inhuman conditions faced by the masses who had been uprooted from the countryside and migrated to overcrowded urban settings, sanitary reformers allowed them to become a working class. The real innovation was that the pioneering sanitarian legislation was almost all about prevention. Very few of the nineteenth-century public health laws were about health care.

The primary goal of government enforcement of public health policies is to allow everyone to benefit from them. Take the employment of children in factories. In the early twentieth century in the United States, a series of state laws prohibited employers from hiring children. The federal government made child labor illegal in 1938 with the Fair Labor Standards Act. Vaccine mandates have the same goal of protecting the whole population as the laws that prohibit employers from hiring minors. Vaccinated persons not only protect themselves, they also contribute to preventing hospitalizations, deaths, school closures, business bankruptcies, unemployment, a breakdown of the health care system, and all the consequences of a severe, long pandemic. For strategies against specific diseases such as measles or COVID-19 to be effective, everyone, whether they are poor or wealthy, whether they live in a rural area or in a city, whether or not they have health insurance, whether they work full time or part time or even at all must have access to safe procedures. If this doesn't happen, the threat may eventually disappear at some point but at a human cost that would be much higher than if public health policies had been implemented across the entire population.

Let's nail it down: Guaranteeing equitable access is the main motive underlying the coercive intervention of governments for backing public health policies. Most people seek protection from their government and expect to receive this protection. Switzerland is a country in which the government asks its population for feedback on key policy questions through routinely organized popular votes. This form of direct democracy has often favored conservative opinions. In 2020, despite a loud and angry opposition, 62% of voters (among the 66% of voters who participated) supported a law providing the legal basis for a COVID-19 certificate with proof of vaccination, negative test, or immunity through having had the virus, to enter bars, cafes, restaurants, cinemas, museums, sporting events, and face-to-face university classes.[8] It is reasonable to expect similar results elsewhere, including in the United States, because only a minority of the population is opposed to the protections for which public health advocates.

The enforcement component of public health has been historically the most difficult to tolerate. Between the fifteenth and the seventeenth century, Italian boards of health imposed quarantines to curb the spread of the plague, but as soon as the plague disappeared from Western Europe in the first decades of the eighteenth century, the opposition to health controls and regulation grew and prevailed. As historian Carlo M. Cipolla puts it: "The concept and practice of public health were born as a reaction to the plague—and somehow they died when the plague disappeared."[9] Similar scenarios occurred when cholera disappeared at the end of the nineteenth century. Today, mask and vaccine mandates generate a reaction against public health that could be expected given the historical precedents.

I suggest in this book that there can be two preventable causes to the alleged "crisis" undergone by public health during the COVID-19 pandemic.[10] The first is to care just as much about the way a public health mandate is implemented as about the way it is established. The Public Health Approach thrives in a democratic environment in which the public, professionals, grassroots organizations, and political parties can weigh in on the process of policymaking. The second is that the Public Health Approach is often misunderstood. Complying with a public health mandate, rule, or law is an issue of collective protection, but it is also the optimal course of action for individuals and their families. A wider understanding of the principles of the Public Health Approach can foster acceptance of and compliance with a public health mandate. It should also help elect to government positions people who campaign on the number of lives that public health has saved.

Chapter 2

Plague

Historians usually locate the roots of public health policies in the earliest human societies and distinguish its premodern from its modern manifestations. The first step toward modern thinking about public health happened in the seventeenth century.[1]

Had death counts been available before the seventeenth century, population thinking might have been more important then. In the absence of health statistics, only intuition could have led health care practitioners or policymakers to reach an understanding of the population dimension of health. The appendix at the end of this book reviews whether there might have been some precursors of population thinking before the seventeenth century.

This chapter is about the first shift in perspective away from thinking in terms of the health of individuals toward thinking about the health of entire populations. The historical context is the seventeenth century, a time of intercontinental migration. You are probably familiar with well-known historical nodes in these long-term processes. Every US student learns in school that the Pilgrims left England on the *Mayflower* and landed in America in 1620. It was also the time that African captives were first brought to North America in 1619. European readers may be more familiar with Alexandre

Dumas's novels *The Three Musketeers, Twenty Years After,* and *The Vicomte of Bragelonne,* which take place sequentially between 1625 and 1673, that is, in the middle half of the seventeenth century.

The century was still experiencing a series of plagues that had swept through Asia, the Middle East, and Europe along international trade routes. These pandemics began with the Black Death (1346–1353), an epidemic of bubonic plague. The last major outbreak of bubonic plague was recorded in 1721. People who became ill with this plague developed symptoms of infection such as fever, headache, chills, and weakness. Swollen, painful tumors in the neck, armpits, and groin were the signatures of bubonic plague. They were called buboes, from the Greek *boubõn,* which meant groin. They could be painful.[2]

It was not understood then that the plague was caused by infected fleas jumping onto humans from the black rats that infested the cramped and dirty streets of London. The dominant idea was that plagues were caused by some form of air pollution, referred to as miasmas, that was released by natural disasters. Some blamed the plague on earthquakes, believing that they released poisonous gases. Earthquakes did precede some plague outbreaks and it is possible that they disturbed rodent populations, causing them to come into closer contact with humans.

The plague traveled through regions that were either next to each other or were linked by trading ships. Noticing the link between ships and outbreaks of plague, some governments began keeping vessels offshore for several weeks when they came from plague-ridden areas. The most common policy was a 40-day embargo, which became known as quarantine, from *quaranta,* the Italian for the number forty. Off-shore embargoes were a pragmatic response to a scourge of unknown origin. They may have given local authorities time to see whether new cases of plague would appear and which lesions could become sources of miasmas.[3]

Quarantining at home became a key component of the response to plague outbreaks. The historian Kira L. S. Newman has described the progression of the plague of 1636 in the London parish of St. Martin-in-the-Fields.[4] In the 1630s, the parish had an unusually high number of boarding houses and bordellos, but many wealthy people also lived in a different part of the parish. It had an estimated population of 10,000, of which 20% were poor receiving assistance from the parish. In October 1635, senior advisors to the king ordered a quarantine of infected ships from France and the Low Countries. However, the quarantine was not rigorously enforced. Within five months, the epidemic had reached London. Within eight months, it had reached St. Martin-in-the-Fields, which was located beyond the city walls. Each parish was responsible for enforcing quarantine and for providing aid and food to quarantined households and individuals. In June 1636, the month the plague reached St. Martin-in-the-Fields, parish officials began to quarantine individual houses. The number of quarantined houses in the parish reached a peak in the fall of 1636, and the policy continued through the first half of 1637. All told, 5,367 people were quarantined during the epidemic; this number represented more than half the population of St. Martin-in-the-Fields. The parish hired nurses to care for the sick and doorkeepers to ensure that no one entered or left quarantined houses. Parish officials also began to incarcerate individuals in pesthouses. This was seen as a stricter means of plague control than quarantining in private homes. The poor were most affected by the plague, but they were not the only ones.

Had the parishes evaluated the impact of their quarantine policies, they would most likely have found them ineffective in preventing the spread of plague because they could not stop the migration of the rats and their fleas. Moreover, these policies could not be rigorously enforced; people bribed or tricked their nurses or doorkeepers. Quarantining was a controversial policy that disrupted social and commercial life and restricted healthy people's access to food, drink, and medical care for forty days.

City officials realized that plague outbreaks usually followed a pattern. Once plague entered a harbor or a town, it spread gradually. After an interval during which there were no deaths, isolated deaths would occur in small clusters in the poorest parishes. These were the harbingers of a scourge that would soon reach all parishes. Wealthy people, politicians, magistrates, and even doctors fled from cities with each return of the pandemic. Soldiers were also safely sheltered in the countryside. Plague outbreaks could thus be extremely disruptive to political and economic life. In some cases, administrative and political institutions were paralyzed because there were no officials left in the city to quell rioting. Thus, plague typically led to social chaos, especially when deserted businesses, houses, and farms began to attract looters. Administrative and political institutions were overwhelmed.

Data and Science

Plague Monitoring

The history of plague recording goes back to the Black Death. From the fourteenth to the seventeenth centuries, churches or city governments (or sometimes both) in Europe formally recorded births, marriages, and deaths. Government officials and wealthy people realized that specifying the cause of death could alert them to an impending outbreak of plague. Having this knowledge in advance could enable the elite to organize a less chaotic retreat from cities.

Italian city-states began to track plague deaths in the mid-fifteenth century. The identification of death from plague was made by a physician, often based on someone else's report rather than on the basis of direct examination of the corpse. These plague rolls are the earliest form of plague recordkeeping. These lists of the names of persons believed to have died from plague did not include a formal count. Entries could be counted up, of course, but neither the physicians who compiled the records nor the government officials who used them would have considered any two individuals as equivalent, even in death. Social rank was carefully recorded because it was an essential consideration for social policy. Even amid massive death and disease, European officials found it impossible to view a beggar, a shopkeeper, a gentleman, and an earl to be units of a same population that could be counted together. The plague rolls listed sick individuals, who were not considered as a group. The plague rolls did not yet allow a shift toward thinking of public health at the population level.

In the 1540s, Henry VIII ordered London officials to compile mortality reports to track the spread of plague. He was the first English monarch to do so during an epidemic. Henry mandated weekly mortality counts in each parish in England and Wales.[5] The reports of the City of London listed all deaths, not just those caused by plague. These data were recorded using Roman numerals. In the mid-1550s, the city established a permanent program to collect a weekly count of every death from each parish together with "how many had died, and whereof they died."[6] Until the plague of 1592, the data were sequestered in government reports. At the height of that outbreak, the city's printer began to post weekly announcements of mortality counts by parish, both from plague and from all causes.[7]

Some parish mortality reports began using arabic numerals in 1603 but generalized that practice only in 1626, when the London Company of Parish Clerks acquired its own printing press. The company's weekly publications reported the death count by parish and also for London overall by cause of death, such as ague (flu), dropsy (heart conditions), suicide, and murder. Although the original manuscript reports of the parish clerks contained many more causes of death than the printed versions, cause of death data in the latter was compiled in a smaller number of categories. Parish clerks also published a summary bill of mortality each year at Christmas. In 1629, the bills began to include the number of christenings, that is, the number of births of Christian children, by gender. The reason for this expansion of content is not known. It may have been related to technical changes that enabled a printer to fit more information on a sheet of paper.

Parish matrons known as searchers collected cause of death data. These women were responsible for visiting the homes of those who had died to determine the cause of death. Their information was based on the report of a relative of the deceased or a physician who had attended the deceased or on their own visual inspection of the corpse.[8] They reported their determinations to the local parish clerk, who then reported the information to the central clerk of his guild. The central clerk compiled a written report for the entire city that was sent to London's mayor and aldermen. He also sent copies to the king and the chancellor. The bills of mortality played a decisive role in the birth of population sciences because they made available a series of quantitative health data that were collected in a relatively similar way over many decades. They provided the platform for a shift to population thinking in public health.

Francis Bacon's Vision

Several profound social changes that took place in the seventeenth century, in addition to the bills, were preconditions of the shift in perspective from individuals to populations. The most obvious is the scientific revolution, which created interest in and an audience for compilations and analyses of empirical data. In Britain, Francis Bacon (1561–1626) advocated the groundbreaking scientific method of tabulating data.[9] In contrast to the speculative approaches to knowledge that had dominated medical theories for centuries, Bacon's method presented information about the presence or absence of a phenomenon in tables and inferred knowledge from analyzing the data in the table.

TABLE 2.1.

Correspondence between Bacon's "images" and observational research biases

BACON'S LATIN	TRANSLATION	MODERN NAMES
Idolum	Image, phantasm	Bias
Idola tribus	False images specific to the human race	Inaccurate observation, information bias, spurious associations
Idola specus	Idiosyncratic images	Preconceived ideas, wish bias
Idola fori	False images emanating from public encounters	Miscommunication and misnomers
Idola theatri	False images resulting from dogmatism	Biased analysis

Bacon also introduced the concept of observational bias. He pointed out that inaccuracies could exist in the collection, tabulation, and analysis of data because of human error. Francis Bacon called these biases "idola," the plural of the Latin *idolum*, "the false appearances that are imposed upon us by the general nature of the mind."[10] Table 2.1 lists the categories of error Bacon identified and their modern equivalents in data science.

Bacon's third contribution to data analysis is the concept of longevity as the indicator of the health of a population. In his 1636 book *Historia vitae et mortae* (*Accounts of Life and Death*),[11] Bacon proposed a research program aimed at identifying the determinants of longevity: these included food, diet, habits of life, exercise, the air in which men live and die, and the places in which people live.[12] Bacon's methodology proved indispensable for a rigorous and meaningful analysis of the bills of mortality by John Graunt.

John Graunt's *Observations*

John Graunt (1620–1674) first published his *Natural and Political Observations on the Bills of Mortality* in 1662, which was not a plague year. The book is often referred to as the *Observations*. Its first edition was an 85-page booklet that included a 19-page appendix. Its twelve chapter headings, listed in Table 2.2, provide a good idea of the mix of natural (related to natural phenomena) and political (social and demographic) factors that Graunt discussed quantitatively using thirty-five years of data drawn from bills of mortality.

Graunt was an accomplished merchant. He and men like him had founded the great commercial and banking houses of the seventeenth and eighteenth centuries.[13] Although he came from a family of merchants and did not have a university education, he

TABLE 2.2.

Chapters of the first edition of Graunt's *Natural and Political Observations on the Bills of Mortality* (1662)

1. Of the Bills of Mortality, their beginning, and progress
2. General Observations upon the Casualties
3. Of Particular Casualties
4. Of the Plague
5. Other Observations upon the Plague, and Casualties
6. Of the Sickliness, Healthfulness, and Fruitfulness of Seasons
7. Of the difference between Burials, and Christenings
8. Of the difference between the numbers of Males, and Females
9. Of the growth of the City
10. Of the Inequality of Parishes
11. Of the number of Inhabitants
12. Of the Country-Bills
The Conclusion

had considerable culture, had studied Latin and French, and could perform the often-complex mathematical operations his business account books required.[14]

Graunt saw an analogy between the contents of the bills of mortality and the double-entry accounting method he used for his business. This method, which was designed to track the stability of profits, required one column of entries for business credits (income and other assets) and one column for debits (payments the business made to vendors and debt holders). The total of these columns should be the same if the accounting is done correctly. The advantage of this system of accounting is that it highlights differences between the two columns of entries so they can be investigated and corrected.[15] Graunt understood that the counts of births and deaths in the City of London's bills of mortality provided a kind of accounting that was analogous to the gains and losses recorded in business accounts and that it was possible to analyze the reported counts to reveal the stability of the ratios of credits (births) to debits (deaths) across time and attempt to explain any irregularities.[16]

Graunt went to the hall of the Company of Parish Clerks and examined the bills of mortality. He summarized the contents of thousands of weekly bills in a set of tables (fig. 2.1). The tables helped him and later others visualize large bodies of data at once, particularly comparisons of births and deaths across years, seasons, parishes, or other divisions of the city.

Using Bacon's approach, Graunt assessed the data for potential biases resulting from how it was collected. There were reasons for concern. The searchers were uneducated elderly women. They were not physicians with the subject matter expertise required to ascertain if someone had died from a specific illness. Smallpox, accident, murder, or suicide could be obvious causes for a layperson

FIGURE 2.1. (*overleaf*) "Table of Casualties" from John Graunt's *Observations and Political Observations Made upon the Bills of Mortality* (1662).

The Years of our Lord	1647	1648	1649	1650	1651	1652	1653	1654	1655	1656	1657	1658	1659
Abortive and Stil-born	335	329	327	351	389	381	384	433	483	419	463	467	421
Aged	916	835	889	696	780	834	864	974	743	892	869	1176	909
Ague and Fever	1260	884	751	970	1038	1212	282	1371	689	875	999	1800	2303
Apoplex and Suddenly	68	74	64	74	106	111	118	86	92	102	113	138	91
Bleach			1	3	7	2				1			
Blasted	4	1			6	6			4		5	5	3
Bleeding	3	2	5	1	3	4	3	2	7	3	5	4	7
Bloody Flux, Scouring and Flux	155	176	802	289	833	762	200	386	168	368	362	233	346
Burnt and Scalded	3	6	10	5	11	8	5	7	10	5	7	4	6
Calenture	1			1		2	1	1			3		
Cancer, Gangrene and Fistula	26	29	31	19	31	53	36	37	73	31	24	35	63
Wolf				8									
Canker, Sore-mouth and Thrush	66	28	54	42	68	51	53	72	44	81	19	27	73
Child-bed	161	106	114	117	206	213	158	192	177	201	236	225	226
Chrisoms and Infants	1369	1254	1065	990	1237	1280	1050	1343	1089	1393	1162	1144	858
Colick and Wind	103	71	85	82	76	102	80	101	85	120	113	179	116
Cold and Cough							41	36	21	58	30	31	33
Consumption and Cough	2423	2200	2388	1988	2350	2410	2286	2868	2606	3184	2757	3610	2982
Convulsion	684	491	530	493	569	653	606	828	702	1027	807	841	742
Cramp			1										
Cut of the Stone		2			1		1	2	4	1	3	5	6
Dropsie and Tympany	185	434	421	508	444	556	617	704	660	706	631	931	646
Drowned	47	40	30	27	49	50	53	30	43	49	63	60	(57
Excessive drinking			2										
Executed	8	17	29	43	24	12	19	21	19	22	20	18	7
Fainted in a Bath				1									
Falling-Sickness	3	2	2	3		3	4	1	4	3	1		4
Flox[1] and small Pox	139	400	1190	184	525	1279	139	812	1294	823	835	409	1523
Found dead in the Streets	6	6	9	8	7	9	14	4	3	4	9	11	2
French-Pox	18	29	15	18	21	20	20	20	29	23	25	53	51
Frighted	4	4	1		3		2		1	1			
Gout	9	5	12	9	7	7	5	6	8	7	8	13	14
Grief	12	13	16	7	17	14	11	17	10	13	10	12	13
Hanged, and made-away themselves	11	10	13	14	9	14	15	9	14	16	24	18	11
Head-Ach			1	11	2		2	6	6	5	3	4	35
Jaundice	57	35	39	49	41	43	57	71	61	41	46	77	102
Jaw-faln	1	1			3			2	2		3	1	
Impostume	75	61	65	59	80	105	79	90	92	122	80	134	105
Itch			1										
Killed by several Accidents	27	57	39	94	47	45	57	58	52	43	52	47	55
King's Evil	27	26	22	19	22	20	26	26	27	24	23	28	28
Lethargy	3	4	2	4	4	4	3	10	9	4	6	2	6
Leprosie			1									1	
Liver-grown, Spleen and Rickets	53	46	56	59	65	72	67	65	52	50	38	51	8
Lunatick	12	18	6	11	7	11	9	12	6	7	13	5	14
Meagrom	12	13		5	8	6	6	14	3	6	7	6	5
Measles	5	92	3	33	33	62	8	52	11	153	15	80	6
Mother	2						1	1	2	2	3	3	
Murdered	3	2	7	5	4	3	3	3	9	6	5	7	70
Overlaid and Starved at Nurse	25	22	36	28	28	29	30	36	58	53	44	50	46
Palsie	27	21	19	20	23	20	29	18	22	23	20	22	17
Plague	3597	611	67	15	23	16	6	16	9	6	4	14	36
Plague in the Guts					1		110	32		87	315	446	253
Pleurisie	30	26	13	20	23	19	17	23	10	9	17	16	12
Poisoned		3		7									
Purples and Spotted Fever	145	47	43	65	54	60	75	89	56	52	56	126	368
Quinsie and Sore-throat	14	11	12	17	24	20	18	9	15	13	7	10	21
Rickets	150	224	216	190	260	329	229	372	347	458	317	476	441
Mother, rising of the Lights	150	92	115	120	134	138	135	178	166	212	203	228	210
Rupture	16	7	7	6	7	16	7	15	11	20	19	18	12
Scal'd head	2					1				2			
Scurvy	32	20	21	21	29	43	41	44	103	71	82	82	95
Smothered and stifled			2										
Sores, ulcers, broken and bruised	15	17	17	16	26	32	25	32	23	34	40	47	61
Shot (Limbs													7
Spleen	12	17					13	13		6	2	5	7
Shingles													1
Starved		4	8	7	1	2	1	1	3	1	3	6	7
Stitch				1		1							
Stone and Strangury	45	42	29	28	50	41	44	38	49	57	72	69	22
Sciatica													
Stopping of the Stomach	29	29	30	33	55	67	66	107	94	145	129	277	186
Surfet	217	137	136	123	104	177	178	212	128	161	137	218	202
Swine-Pox	4	4	3			1	4	2	1	1		1	2
Teeth and Worms	767	597	540	598	709	905	691	1131	803	1198	878	1036	839
Tissick	62	47											
Thrush											57	66	
Vomiting	1	6	3	7	4	6	3	14	7	27	16	19	8
Worms	147	107	105	65	85	86	53						
Wen	1		1		2	2				1		2	1
Suddenly													

660	1629	1630	1631	1632	1633	1634	1635	1636	1629 1630 1631 1632	1633 1634 1635 1636	1647 1648 1649 1650	1651 1652 1653 1654	1655 1656 1657 1658	1629 1649 1659	In 20 Years.
544	499	439	410	445	500	475	507	523	1793	2005	1342	1587	1832	1247	8559
095	579	712	661	671	704	623	794	714	2475	2814	3336	3452	3680	2377	15759
148	956	1091	1115	1108	953	1279	1622	2360	4418	6235	3865	4903	4363	4010	23784
67	22	36		17	24	35	26		75	85	280	421	445	177	1306
									4		4	9	1	1	15
8	13	8	10	13	6	4		4	54	14	5	12	14	16	99
2	5	2	5	4	4	3			16	7	11	12	19	17	65
251	449	438	352	348	278	512	346	330	1587	1466	1422	2181	1161	1597	7818
6	3	10	7	5	1	3	12	3	25	19	24	31	26	19	125
							1	3		4	2	4	3		13
52	20	14	23	28	27	30	24	30	85	112	105	157	150	114	609
										8					8
68	6	4	4	1			5	74	15	79	190	244	161	133	689
194	150	157	112	171	132	143	163	230	590	668	498	769	839	490	3304
123	2596	2378	2035	2268	2130	2315	2113	1895	9277	8453	4678	4910	4788	4519	32106
167	48	57					37	50	105	87	341	359	497	247	1389
24	10	58	51	55	45	54	50	57	174	207	00	77	140	43	598
414	1827	1910	1713	1797	1754	1955	2080	2477	5157	8266	8999	9914	12157	7197	44487
031	52	87	18	241	221	386	418	709	498	1734	2198	2656	3377	1324	9073
			1	0	0	0	0	0	01	00	01	0	0	1	2
4				5	1	5	2	2	5	10	6	4	13	47	38
872	235	252	279	280	266	250	329	389	1048	1734	1538	2321	2982	1302	9623
48)	43	33	29	34	37	32	32	45	139	147	144	182	215	130	827
											2			2	2
18	19	13	12	18	13	13	13	13	62	52	97	76	79	55	384
											1				1
5	3	10	7	7	2	5	6	8	27	21	10	8	8	9	74
354	72	40	58	531	72	1354	293	127	701	1846	1913	2755	3361	2785	10576
6	18	33	20	6	13	8	24	24	83	69	29	34	27	29	243
31	17	12	12	12	7	17	12	22	53	48	80	81	130	83	392
								3	2	3	9	5	2	2	21
9	1			1				8	8						
2	2	5	3	4	4	5	7		14	24	35	25	36	28	134
4	18	20	22	11	14	17	5	20	71	56	48	59	45	47	279
36	8	8	6	15		3	8	7	37	18	48	47	72	32	222
26							4	2	0	6	14	14	17	46	051
76	47	59	35	43	35	45	54	63	184	197	180	212	225	188	998
	10	16	13	8	10	10	4	11	47	35	02	5	6	10	95
96	58	76	73	74	50	62	73	130	282	315	260	35	428	228	1639
					10				00	10	01				11
47	54	55	47	46	49	41	51	60	202	201	217	207	194	148	1021
54	16	25	18	38	35	20	20	69	97	150	94	94	102	66	537
4	1		2	2	3		2	2	5	7	13	21	21	9	67
2	2						2	2	2	2	1		1	3	06
15	94	12	99	87	82	77	98	99	392	356	213	269	191	158	1421
14	6	11	6	5	4	2	2	5	28	13	47	39	31	26	158
4			24				22	22	24	22	30	34	22	05	132
74	42	2	3	80	21	33	27	12	127	83	133	155	259	51	757
8	1						3	3	01	3	2	4	8	02	18
20			3	7		6	5	8	10	19	17	13	27	77	86
43	4	10	13	7	8	14	10	14	34	46	111	123	215	86	529
21	17	23	17	25	14	21	25	17	82	77	87	90	87	53	423
14		1317	274	8		1		10400	1599	10401	4290	61	33	103	16384
402									00	00	61	142	844	253	991
10	26	24	26	36	21		45	24	112	90	89	72	52	51	415
					2			2	2	00	4	10	00	00	14
146	32	58	58	38	24	125	245	397	186	791	300	278	290	243	1845
14	01	8	6	7	24	04	5	22	22	55	54	71	45	34	247
521						14	49	50	00	113	780	1190	1598	657	3681
249	44	72	99	98	60	84	72	104	309	220	777	585	809	369	2700
28	2	6	4	9	4	3	10	13	21	30	36	45	68	21	201
											2	1	2		05
12	5	7	9		9		00	25	33	34	94	132	300	115	593
		24							24		2			2	26
48	23		20	48	19	19	22	29	91	89	65	115	144	141	504
20														07	27
7											29	26	13	07	68
					1					1				1	2
14									14		19	5	13	29	51
											1				1
30	35	39	58	50	58	49	33	45	114	185	144	173	247	51	937
2				1	3		1	6	1	4					13
214								6		6	121	295	247	216	669
192	63	157	149	86	104	114	132	371	445	721	613	671	644	401	3094
	5	8	4	6	3		10		23	13	11	5	5	10	57
008	440	506	335	470	432	454	539	1207	1751	2632	2502	3436	3915	1819	14236
8	8	12	14	34	23	15	27		68	65	109			8	242
	15	23	17	40	28	31	34		95	93			123	15	211
10	1	4	1	1	2	5	6	3	7	16	17	27	69	12	136
	19	31	28	27	19	28	27		105	74	424	224		124	830
1			1		4				1	4	2	4	4	2	15
	63	59	37	62	58	62	78	34	221	233				63	454
														34190	229250

but not all were. Moreover, the searchers worked with no supervision and were suspected of being open to bribery and coercion by relatives who wanted to avoid quarantine because a household member had died of plague or who wanted to avoid the stigma associated with certain causes of death, such as venereal diseases.

Could the bills be trusted, Graunt asked, given that they reported the conclusions of searchers who likely made errors? There were many reasons that the reports of some searchers might be inaccurate or unreliable. Nonetheless, Graunt reasoned, searchers identified diseases and other causes of death based on observable signs and symptoms, and that did not require more knowledge than an ordinary person had. For example, identifying a cause of death as grief, drowning, or suicide ("men making away with themselves") required only common sense. Moreover, the city had empowered its searchers to consult anyone who could help them arrive at a cause, including physicians who were familiar with the deceased. Indeed, the patterns in the data and the stability of the numbers reported suggested that despite the possibility of errors in particular cases, the searchers' reports were trustworthy. In his own analysis, Graunt was careful to guard against overinterpretation of the trends in causes of death that required medical expertise to determine.

Astonishing Regularities

Using the double-entry accounting method, Graunt examined the stability of the searchers' reported counts across time. He discovered that although the exact numbers varied across time, the annual number of deaths from all causes (except plague) in the City of London seemed to be 7,000 to 8,000 (except for plague years). The stability of mortality counts in epidemic-free years was unexpected. Until that point, it was impossible to predict how many people would die in a given year. Yet the bills of mortality suggested that 7,000 to 8,000 people would die in any given year.

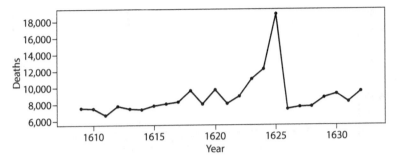

FIGURE 2.2. Number of deaths from all causes except the plague in London, 1609–1632; data from *John Graunt's Observations and Political Observations Made upon the Bills of Mortality* (1662).

Because there were no censuses then, the size of London's population was unknown. However, it is fair to assume that it grew slowly and regularly. The city had a limited number of dwellings, paid positions, and beds, and the attractions of London life were such that each time a position became free, a fresh migrant from the countryside filled it. The stability of the numbers across time made any deviation in that pattern suspect. For example, the records clearly misreported the expected mortalities in 1625, a plague year. Figure 2.2 depicts the compiled numbers of death from all causes but the plague from 1609 to 1632. Across that period, 7,000 to 8,000 persons died each year, except for 1625, when 18,848 people died from causes other than the plague, almost 11,000 more than expected. Graunt suggested that inaccurate reports from the searchers could be an explanation for this outlier data in 1625, which was one of the worst plague years of the century in London. It may be that overwhelmed searchers were not able to identify plague as the correct cause for many of those 11,000 excess deaths.

The Consequential Switch

Deaths from specific causes fell into two major patterns in the bills of mortality. Epidemic diseases such plague, smallpox, and measles

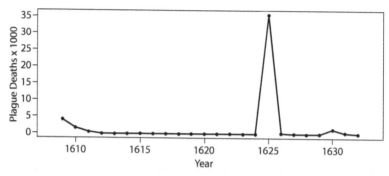

FIGURE 2.3. Number of deaths from the plague in London, 1609–1632; data from John Graunt's *Observations and Political Observations Made upon the Bills of Mortality* (1662).

caused deaths at irregular intervals. There had been almost no reported casualties from the plague for several years before and after the severe outbreak of 1625 (fig. 2.3).

Even during an outbreak, the number of casualties from epidemic diseases fluctuated enormously. The number of plague deaths, for example, could jump in one week from 118 to 927, then back to 258 the next week and up to 852 the week after that. Epidemics were acute and irregular events.[17] A second type of disease tended to account for a "constant proportion" of the overall mortality. Graunt called these causes of death "chronic diseases."[18] They included consumption (mostly tuberculosis), dropsy (most likely edema from congestive heart failure), jaundice, gout, stone, palsy, scurvy, rickets, different forms of fevers, and accidents. This category of causes accounted for 80% of all London deaths.

"Consumption and cough," most likely from tuberculosis, accounted for about 22% of all deaths excluding plague deaths in the period 1628 to 1660 (fig. 2.4). There is a gap in the data for 1637 to 1646 because Graunt found the decade "uninformative" and omitted it from all his analyses. We don't know why he dropped these ten years and can only speculate that he did not believe that exam-

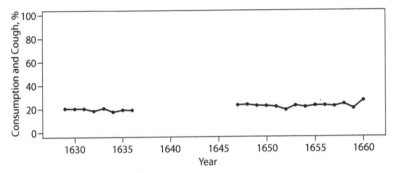

FIGURE 2.4. Proportion of deaths from all causes (except the plague) due to consumption and cough in London, 1629–1636 and 1647–1660; data from John Graunt's *Observations and Political Observations Made upon the Bills of Mortality* (1662).

ining them would reveal anything new. Keep in mind that reporting the results of a decade of data involved copying and compiling the information from up to 520 weekly bills plus the annual summaries, all of which had to be done by hand using a quill pen and ink. That was quite an endeavor in the seventeenth century.

Distinguishing between acute diseases, which caused numbers of death that fluctuated across time, and chronic diseases, which caused a constant portion of all deaths, provided information about the state of health of the population of London, conceived, to use the metaphor I proposed in the preface, as a superindiviual. Graunt wrote that chronic diseases indicated the "ordinary temper of the place," the "fitness of the country for long life," and "the wholesomeness of the food."[19] He deemed a country with a larger proportion of deaths from chronic disease than other countries to be sicklier and said that its population would likely live shorter lives.

In his analysis of the bills of mortality, Graunt discovered that switching the perspective from thinking in terms of individuals to thinking in terms of a population provided a wealth of knowledge about health, disease, and death that had seemed beyond the reach of human intelligence.

Plague Vanishes

The irregularity of losses from plague suggested that the epidemic had an environmental origin. Graunt believed that plague was transmitted via some form of air pollution. This was a common belief of the time. The Black Death of the fourteenth century and its subsequent periodic recurrence were thought to have been originally unleashed by a deadly corruption of the air. It was believed that people who breathed the corrupted air fell sick. Physicians who attended patients often wore masks with long leather beaks that held dried flowers and other odoriferous plants under their noses to neutralize the smell of fetid air.

The *Observations* first appeared in January 1662, about two years after Charles II ascended to the throne in May 1660. The fact that it was written in English rather than Latin meant that citizens and public officials could read it, not just rulers. In the aftermath of the Restoration of the English monarchy, Graunt intended his book to help the government better manage social issues and issues related to health using what we would call today evidence.[20] For example, his analysis of the bills of mortality debunked the astrology-based belief that great plagues occurred with each major political transition. There had been plagues in 1603 after the coronation of James I and in 1625, after the coronation of Charles I, but not after Charles was beheaded in 1648 or after the restoration of the monarchy in 1660. Indeed, 1648 and 1660 were markedly healthful and fecund years. Instead, Graunt's analysis of the bills of mortality suggested that quarantining water-borne vessels and migrants to the city could help control the plague because it seemed to have spread due to environmental causes that were not permanently present in the City of London. The *Observations* could thus foster good governance if political parties and factions within church and state could agree about what the data said and find common ground before passing new laws.

Graunt wrote that by comparing the number of casualties from a specific cause to the mortality from all causes, Londoners could "better understand the hazard they are in."[21] In modern language, they could assess their risk of dying from various causes. Londoners were interested in predictions about health. They were avid consumers of astrological predictions about the course and destiny of human affairs. Long before risks could be calculated using mortality data, people referred to astrological predictions in almanacs that were typically published each year. Almanacs of the seventeenth century used astrology to predict the occurrence of natural phenomena such as the effect of weather on agriculture or the course of epidemics of venereal diseases.[22] Astrologist John Gadbury used the positions of planets in the sky in 1665 to predict the growth and decline of the plague that year.[23] Such predictions were common across not just Europe but also in China, India, and the Mediterranean. Londoners who read the bills of mortality and Graunt's *Observations*, however, were the first human beings who had epidemiological insights into their future health.

At the urging of his friend William Petty, Graunt presented copies of the *Observations* to the king and his chief ministers and sent fifty copies to the Royal Society of London, which almost immediately proposed him as a candidate for membership. After the king had personally recommended him and a committee of the society had examined *Observations*, Graunt was elected to the prestigious society on February 26, 1662.[24]

The *Observations* rapidly went through several editions. A second edition was issued within a year of the first. Three more editions were published over the next fifteen years, including one brought out just after Graunt's death in 1674. There were also many copycat publications and commentaries by other writers who hoped to cash in on the popularity of the book.

By an interesting coincidence, last great epidemic London's took place in 1665, three years after the first edition of the *Observations*, even though major outbreaks continued on the continent of Europe for another sixty years. British medicine could not have contributed to such an outcome, as British doctors had no effective treatments or preventive measures. Germ theory would not be developed for two centuries, and the role of fleas from rats and that of the bacterium *Yersinia pestis* in the transmission of plague were not yet understood (Alexandre Yersin discovered the cause of plague in 1894). Could the disappearance of the plague in London be related in any way to the publication of Graunt's book? Some historians have stressed the role of quarantine and police or military control of infected areas that prevented anyone from leaving them, the so-called *cordons sanitaires*, after 1662 (that is, immediately after the first publication of the *Observations*).[25] For example, in 1663, the first English quarantine regulations required ships with suspected infected passengers or crew to remain in the estuary of the River Thames. However, there are several other plausible explanations for the disappearance of the plague from London. Brown rats, which are less susceptible to fleas, may have replaced black rats. After the Great Fire of London in 1665, many houses were built with brick rather than wood. This separated humans from their domestic animals more effectively and limited the circulation of rats in the dwelling areas of houses.[26]

Graunt's Accomplishment

In the appendix, I argue that there was no evidence of rigorous, modern public health thinking at the level of populations before the seventeenth century. There is a consensus that the *Observations* are the common ancestor of all population-based sciences such as statistics, epidemiology, sociology, and demography.[27]

Graunt was aware that he had done something new. He wrote that he had had "much pleasure in deducing so many abstruse, and unexpected inferences out of these poor despised Bills of Mortality."[28]

It would be incorrect, however, to think that he was solely responsible for initiating the Public Health Approach. There were scientific, political, and technical reasons for the emergence of that approach.

Scientific. The *Observations* were an explicit attempt to apply Bacon's new methodology to the analysis of fifty years' worth of birth and mortality data collected in London. Francis Bacon influenced Graunt in at least three domains: tabulating data, discussing the accuracy of the parish searchers' reports in terms of some of the biases Bacon described, and identifying the determinants of longevity.

Political. A decisive step occurred in 1603, when King James allowed the London Company of Parish Clerks to print the bills of mortality on a weekly basis. The collection of data about a series of health events that occurred across time revealed patterns of occurrence that could not have been suspected otherwise.

Technical. The collection of data for and eventual printing of the bills of mortality required an administrative infrastructure. The City of London, its parishes, and the Company of Parish Clerks jointly provided that infrastructure. The parishes enrolled matrons to visit homes where a death had occurred. A matron who had been chosen as a searcher was sworn to uphold her duty as a city official and was issued a wand as a public mark of her authority. The parish also paid her a small fee. Because of their age, it is likely that the searchers had acquired immunity to some diseases. They were familiar with the lifestyles of many in their parish and had become experienced in recognizing immediate causes of death in children and adults. They reported to their parish clerks, who registered counts at the parish level and transmitted them to the clerk of the Company of Parish Clerks, who transcribed them and sent a summary to the aldermen of the City of London. The clerk of the guild also sent copies to the king and his chancellor. Parish clerks issued an annual summary bill each year at Christmas. All of these documents were bound and stored at the hall of the Company of Parish Clerks, although many were destroyed in fires over the centuries.

The *Observations* were thus preconditioned by an extraordinary set of circumstances. The seventeenth century ended with the first work that can unquestionably be considered a solid foundation for the Public Health Approach.

Chapter 3

Smallpox

The decline in mortality from smallpox in the Western world began in the eighteenth century, thanks to variolation, the ancestor of the first vaccine. It usually consisted in inoculating under the skin of persons who had never had smallpox a small amount of pus from someone else's variolous pustules. Assessing the efficacy of variolation to immunize against a natural infection of smallpox featured a pioneering implementation of an essential principle of the Public Health Approach which had been missing against the plague: efficacy of interventions can be proved by comparing groups of people. Group comparisons conferred a scientific foundation on the Public Health Approach.

The last major outbreaks of bubonic plague in Western Europe began in 1720. The disappearance of plague shifted the focus to smallpox, a disease that had caused 25% of all deaths in London during the seventeenth century. It also left terrible scars on the faces and bodies of those who survived it.[1]

The Greatest Killer

Smallpox is caused by the variola virus. The disease typically began with symptoms such as high fever, headache, and pain in the back and muscles. The flu-like symptoms were followed by a pox, red spots on the skin and mucosae. Within a few days, some of the spots would become blisters (papules, or poxes) that were filled with a clear serum and, after a few more days, with pus. The virus lived within the contents of the blisters. Poxes spread over the entire body but occurred most densely on the face, arms, and legs. In lethal cases, the poxes fused. The exudations from the papules had a terrible smell. Papules evolved into scabs that fell off and left permanently disfigured faces and pitted skin over large areas of the body. Blindness and sometimes male infertility could result.

Smallpox could be spread by objects contaminated by the content of the papules, such as bedding or clothing, which created great risk for the people who cared for patients. However, epidemics occurred mostly because of airborne transmission. When the contagious papules appeared in the mouths and throats of patients, the virus spread when those patients coughed or sneezed.[2]

Originally an animal disease, smallpox adapted to humans more than 4,000 years ago after the advent of a more sedentary lifestyle that included agriculture and animal husbandry.[3] Over the following 2,000 years it emerged in a few centers of unusually dense human population in Egypt, India, China, and Greece,[4] then spread into the Mediterranean. About 1,000 years ago, almost every adult alive in Asia and Europe had survived the infection and was immune to subsequent exposure. Children, the main pool of susceptible hosts, suffered greatly; smallpox had become a childhood disease. Before Columbus, smallpox was unknown in the New World, but it became one of the diseases (along with measles and flu) that Europeans and Africans brought to the Americas. In the fifteenth and sixteenth centuries, these diseases wiped out 90% of the 50 to 100 million Indigenous people of the Caribbean and Central America.[5] Smallpox ravaged North American Indian tribes from the early seventeenth century to the end of the nineteenth century.[6]

Deaths from smallpox began to be monitored in England in the seventeenth century. British physicians were not used yet to refer to the bills of mortality to assess its prevalence. They made best guesses, as when the English physician Thomas Sydenham wrote, "The Small pox of all other diseases is the most common, as that which sooner or later (at least in this part of the world) attaques most men."[7] The use of "most" to characterize the prevalence of the disease is typical of ancient Western medicine since Hippocrates, as I show in the appendix of this book. In contrast, the bills of mortality indicate that London was hit by a severe epidemic of smallpox approximately every three years. During the 22 years recorded by John Graunt, and shown in figure 2.1, there had been 12,453 deaths from "flox and smallpox" (5% of all deaths) and 16,433 from the plague (7% of all deaths). By 1700, the disease was endemic among both the wealthy and the poor in large cities of more than 200,000 inhabitants worldwide.[8]

Eighteenth-century doctors viewed smallpox as the result of a process analogous to fermentation that they believed took place in the blood. This was consistent with their speculative theories that good health required a balancing of the four humors of the body. Fermentation, doctors believed, raised a person's temperature and released its poisonous scum in pustules. They told their patients to avoid hot food that would increase fermentation. They used emetics and enemas to purge the bodies of smallpox patients of corrupt materials in their stomach and bowel. Medical opinions diverged as to whether patients should be bled and whether they should be kept in a warm or cold environment.[9]

A controversy erupted around 1700 in Britain and America about the efficacy of inoculating people with smallpox pus, a folk practice in much of Asia, Arabia, North Africa, India, and Turkey.[10] In China, an elaborate method of inoculation involved inserting swabs of cotton with infected pus in a nostril. In Turkey, women put tiny amounts of variolous material under the skin of children, that is, inoculated the disease. In 1717, Lady Mary Wortley Montague, the wife of the British ambassador to the Sublime Porte, the central government of the Ottoman Empire, wrote a letter from Constantinople (now Istanbul) to a friend that described the local practice of elderly women deliberately inducing a mild form of the disease.[11] Lady Montague had both her children inoculated. Her initiative prompted disputes and research about the safety of the immunization technique on both sides of the Atlantic.

The question was one that could be addressed using population data: Was smallpox created by inoculation more or less lethal than smallpox acquired by natural means? The answer in America and Britain in the 1720s was a groundbreaking step for the Public Health Approach.

Pioneering Group Comparisons
Boston 1721

In early May of 1721, a major epidemic of smallpox hit Boston following the arrival of HMS *Sea Horse* from the West Indies. A few cases were quickly quarantined, and city officials ordered the ship to leave the harbor. The authorities believed that they had dodged the threat, but a week later eight more people became sick. From that point, the contagion grew out of control.

Rev. Cotton Mather, an influential minister, had been convinced by articles in the journal of the Royal Society of London, of which he was a member, that inoculations saved lives. He had also been influenced by Onesimus, an enslaved Guaramantee from southern Libya,[12] who had undergone the procedure in Africa and had been protected from the disease since then. Early in the outbreak, Mather reached out to the medical community of Boston, imploring them to use the inoculation method. One physician, Zabdiel Boylston, heeded his call, but most other doctors were hostile to the idea. At the forefront of the opposition was one of Boston's only practitioners who had a medical degree, William Douglass.

When the epidemic declined in early 1722, about half the city's population had been infected (5,759 people out of around 10,600).[13] According to records, about 8% of Bostonians (844) had succumbed to it from April 1721 to February 1722.[14] The severity of the epidemic can be fathomed by comparing those ratios with the death toll from COVID-19, which killed 0.2% of the US population in 2020, forty times less than the proportion of Boston's population that died from smallpox in those eleven months in 1721 and 1722.

Mather and Boylston made a pioneering comparison using data on the lethality of smallpox as the result of inoculation versus the lethality of naturally contracted smallpox. Only 2% of the 287 people Boylston had inoculated died, while 14.7% (844/ 5,759) of people who were not inoculated and became ill with smallpox during the same period died.[15]

Mather and Boylston did a group comparison that showed that inoculated people were about seven times less likely to die from smallpox than those who were not inoculated and caught the disease. The results were highly consistent with results from other populations that repeatedly showed the benefits of the procedure published in the *Philosophical Transactions of the Royal Society of London*.

However, Mather and Boylston's data did not quell the intense debate about the safety of inoculation the epidemic had generated. The supporters of inoculation were led by Mather and Boylston. Most clergymen in Boston supported Mather's position. When Rev. Mather was criticized for endorsing a secular treatment for disease, thus thwarting God's will, he responded, "Almighty God, in his great Mercy to Mankind, has taught us a Remedy to be used, when the Dangers of the Small Pox distress us."[16]

Those opposed to inoculation were led by William Douglass. He believed that injecting smallpox-filled pus contradicted both the ethical medical principle of "first do no harm" and the Bible's sixth commandment ("Thou shalt not kill"). With the exception of

Boylston, Boston's doctors supported Douglass. Their position was that it was their role to decide which medical procedures were most appropriate; they were angry because they felt that Mather, a clergyman, had usurped this role. Ignoring the publications of the *Philosophical Transactions* and Boylston's data, they were concerned that the technique of infecting healthy persons, which they characterized as untested and based on folk practices, could cause more deaths from the disease. They also feared that smallpox could spread from inoculated patients.[17]

While science and religion figured as support for the views of the two opposing sides in this controversy, both sides also used racist arguments. In 1702, Mather, the clergyman who later argued from the position of scientific evidence, wrote that as a result of smallpox epidemics, "the woods were almost cleared of these pernicious creatures [local Indigenous people], to make room for better growth"[18] Douglass also suggested that inoculation could be used as a weapon to exterminate native Indian populations.

In hindsight, the real watershed moment for public health history was the population thinking of Boylston and Mather, who collected data about two groups, one treated and one untreated. Their evidence confirmed that people who were inoculated had a seven times greater chance of surviving smallpox than people who were not. The physicians who opposed inoculation believed that infecting a healthy person puts that person at risk and can propagate the infection. Thus, for the Boston doctors, the procedure was unethical. Their experience as medical practitioners treating individual patients was insufficient to convince them that the immunizing procedure was safer than the disease.

Saving Lives

The strongest evidence that inoculation was effective was published just a couple of years after the Boston outbreak of 1721–1722. James Jurin (1684–1750), a British doctor who had received his medical training in Leiden, had a mathematical background and had applied Newtonian physics to explore aspects of the physiology of the heart.[19] Jurin wanted to know "whether the Hazard of Inoculation be considerably less than that of the natural Small Pox."[20]

While Jurin was secretary of the Royal Society of London, he conducted a pioneering survey.[21] Thanks to his reputation and his connection to the members of the Royal Society, Jurin was able to gather data from twenty places in Britain where doctors he knew and respected had recorded the number of deaths following smallpox infection among uninoculated people. The lethality from the naturally contracted disease was 16.3%, or one in six.[22]

Obtaining data about people who had been inoculated was more complicated. On December 11, 1723, Jurin published an advertisement in the *Philosophical Transactions of the Royal Society* asking all persons involved with the practice of inoculation to contribute to a register that recorded the name, age, location, mode of inoculation, clinical history, and death or survival of inoculated patients.[23] He received information on 474 cases, of which 440 had the smallpox by inoculation (table 3.1). Five of the inoculated people had an imperfect reaction and 29 had no reaction. Nine of them died. Jurin provided detailed clinical histories of the nine who died. For all but one, there were plausible reasons for the deaths other than inoculation, but for the sake of convincing the anti-inoculation group, Jurin chose the most conservative estimate of mortality, 9 out of 440, or 1.9%. Jurin reported that 1.9% of healthy people who had been inoculated had died and, as mentioned above, 16.3% of uninoculated people who became ill with smallpox died.[24] His data showed that the intervention was much safer than the naturally contracted illness—eight times less lethal, in fact.

The mathematically trained scientist carried the reasoning further, establishing a new use of population thinking. He computed the public health implications of his comparative study. According to the Bills of Mortality, an average of 2,287 people died of smallpox

TABLE 3.1.

Total number of persons reported to James Jurin as having been inoculated by 37 British practitioners in 1721, 1722, 1723 and the outcome of the inoculation

AGES	PERSONS INOCULATED	HAD THE SMALL POX BY INOCULATION	HAD AN IMPERFECT SMALL POX BY INOCULATION	NO EFFECT	SUSPECTED TO HAVE DIED OF INOCULATION
Under 1 year	11	11	0	0	0
1 year to 2	15	14		1	2
2 to 3	31	31	0	0	1
3 to 4	41	38	0	3	1
4 to 5	33	31	0	2	1
5 to 10	140	137	1	02	2
10 to 15	82	76	0	6	0
15 to 20	56	50	1	5	2
20 to 52	62	50	3	9	0
Age unknown	3	2	0	1	0
Total	474	440	5	29	9

Source: J. Jurin, *An Account of the Success of Inoculating the Small Pox in Great Britain: With a Comparison between the Miscarriages in that Practice, and the Mortality of the Natural Small-Pox* (London: Peele, 1724), 17, https://quod.lib.umich.edu/.

every year in London. If—as shown in his survey—the death rate represented one in six people naturally infected, the 2,287 deaths must have resulted from 13,722 sick Londoners ($6 \times 2,287 = 13,722$). Had these 13,722 Londoners been inoculated, only 1.9% of them, or 261 (1.9% of $13,722 = 261$) would have died. Thus, inoculation had the potential to prevent 2,026 deaths ($2,287 - 261 = 2,026$)

each year in London. Jurin concluded: "Consequently 2,000 persons that are yearly cut off, within the Bills of Mortality alone, and those generally in the beginning, or prime of life, might be preserved to their King and country."[25]

From Inoculation to Vaccines

By the late 1750s, inoculation was widely performed by British doctors, country surgeons, and even locally trained apothecaries and amateurs.[26] In North America, the evidence in favor of the procedure converted journalist, scientist, and future diplomat Benjamin Franklin from an opposer of vaccination to an active promoter. During the 1721 epidemic in Boston, he had worked at the newspaper of his brother, James, who printed material that criticized Cotton Mather and Zabdiel Boylston and disparaged their campaigns. However, in 1730, after an epidemic of smallpox struck New England, Franklin published an article in his own journal, the *Pennsylvania Gazette*, that reported that 4% died among those were inoculated compared to 25% of those who were not inoculated. Inoculation, wrote Benjamin Franklin, was a "safe and beneficial practice."[27]

In 1736, when Deborah and Benjamin Franklin's son, Francis Folger, died of smallpox at age 4, rumors circulated that the young boy had contracted the disease through inoculation. Actually, the child had not been inoculated. The procedure had been postponed because of an episode of diarrhea. In his autobiography, Benjamin Franklin stressed the importance of immunizing children:

> In 1736 I lost one of my sons, a fine boy of four years old, by the small-pox, taken in the common way. I long regretted bitterly, and still regret that I had not given it to him by inoculation. This I mention for the sake of parents who omit that operation, on the supposition that they should never forgive themselves if a child died under it, my example

showing that the regret may be the same either way and that, therefore, the safer should be chosen.[28]

In February 1759, Benjamin Franklin wrote the preface for Dr. William Heberden's pamphlet *Some accounts of the success of inoculation for the smallpox in England and America. Together with plain instructions, by which any person may be enabled to perform the operation, and conduct the patient through the distemper.*[29] Franklin's reasoning is important because he built a case in favor of inoculation from observations that seemed to support the anti-inoculation views.

Franklin first reported mortality data from an epidemic of smallpox that occurred in Boston in 1753 or 1754. After a period of confusion, some residents decided to inoculate themselves and their families. In order to assess the efficacy of inoculation, Boston magistrates requested that the constables of each city ward, assisted by both partisans and opponents of the inoculation, perform a "strict and impartial enquiry." Together, officers and their assistants went "through the wards from house to house" and collected data that showed that smallpox had killed 8.9% of uninoculated whites and 12.8% of uninoculated Blacks. In contrast, the mortality rate among inoculated people was only 1.2% among whites and 5% among Blacks.[30]

The mortality rate for inoculated people was lower than that who acquired smallpox from natural infection but still higher than what Franklin expected based on recent data from the London Smallpox Hospital. Franklin suggested that in Boston the "great hurry of business" had led surgeons and physicians to inoculate patients who would not typically have been inoculated because they were too weak or debilitated or were suffering from other illnesses.[31]

Franklin concluded that the evidence still favored inoculation even though it was less than perfect and would still do so "if the chance were only as two to one in favor of the practice among children." The high cost of the procedure may explain why only 30%

of Blacks had been inoculated compared to 40% of whites. Franklin established the Society for Inoculating the Poor Gratis in 1774 to counter this inequity.[32]

Smallpox inoculation may have had strategic implications in the American Revolutionary War.[33] The 1776 Canadian Campaign was brutally interrupted by smallpox. Because of it, the Northern Army had "melted away."[34] In June 1776 John Adams wrote that "The small-pox is ten times more terrible than Britons, Canadians, and Indians together. This was the cause of our precipitate retreat from Quebeck."[35] Had Quebec fallen, it could have entailed the inclusion of great parts of Canada in the American Revolution. On February 6, 1777, the Continental Congress approved a plan to systematically inoculate soldiers.[36] The procedure was implemented over the next two years. As Arthur Boylston has noted, "inoculation became as much a part of soldiering as a musket."[37] Inoculation may well have helped tipped the balance toward the Patriots during the Revolution. The colonial and English armies were unequally susceptible to smallpox. Most British soldiers were immune from previous infection or from inoculation, while George Washington's troops came from rural areas where there was a low prevalence of smallpox. Because of that, they were highly susceptible to the disease. The threat of smallpox disincentivized recruitment into the Continental Army. But after the Continental Army was inoculated, it began to consistently win battles such as Cowpens in 1881 and of course Yorktown.

In other words, the revolution was won because the revolutionaries were "vaxed." However, the term "vaccine" had still to be invented. During the second half of the eighteenth century, some British country doctors noticed that many people working on farms did not develop smallpox when they were inoculated with pus that contained the virus. Typically, these people had previously contracted cowpox (*Variolae vaccinæ*), a benign disease.[38] News of this observation spread and people began to wonder if the very safe artificial inoculation of cowpox could confer immunity against smallpox.

Edward Jenner (1749–1823), a physician in Gloucestershire, was aware of the claims that natural infection of cowpox protected people from contracting smallpox. He tested the procedure on healthy people. His most famous case was that of an eight-year-old boy, James Phipps, whom he selected to receive an inoculum of cowpox from a pustule on the hand of a dairymaid named Sarah Nelmes on May 14, 1796. Phipps suffered from fever and some uneasiness but no great illness. When Phipps was repeatedly injected with material containing the smallpox virus six weeks later, he did not develop a pustule at the inoculation site or the severe symptoms generally associated with variolation. The vaccine (from *vacca*, Latin for cow) was effective.

The Royal Society of London rejected Jenner's manuscript describing one of the most consequential scientific discoveries ever made.[39] The members did not deem the success Jenner achieved with James Phipps to be enough evidence to support the adoption of cowpox inoculation. One example was not convincing; twenty or thirty would have been better.[40] This setback stimulated Jenner to inoculate a series of patients with cowpox followed by inoculation for smallpox, but he chose not to submit a revised text to the Royal Society. Instead, he published a book privately in 1798, *An Inquiry into the Causes and Effects of the Variolae Vaccinae: A Disease Discovered in Some of the Western Counties of England, Particularly Gloucestershire, and Known by the Name of the Cow Pox.* Jenner believed that it would be "unnecessary to produce further testimony" in support of his assertion that "the cow-pox protects the human constitution from the infection of the smallpox."[41]

The discovery of the cowpox vaccine did not require a population approach. Comparing the vaccine to inoculation in different groups was not needed in this case. Effective immunization of a few persons sufficed. Even though inoculation remained a procedure of choice for many doctors for decades, vaccination overcame opposition and progressively became accepted.[42] Smallpox was finally eradicated in the twentieth century thanks to a worldwide vaccination campaign directed by Donald Ainslee Henderson that concluded in 1980.[43] The World Health Assembly commemorated the public health milestone:

> Declaration of Global Eradication of Smallpox
> The Thirty-third World Health Assembly, on this the eighth day of May 1980; Having considered the development and results of the global program on smallpox eradication initiated by WHO in 1956 and intensified since 1967;
> 1. Declares solemnly that the world and all its peoples have won freedom from smallpox, which was a most devastating disease sweeping in epidemic form through many countries since earliest times, leaving death, blindness and disfigurement in its wake and which only a decade ago was rampant in Africa, Asia and South America;
> 2. Expresses its deep gratitude to all nations and individuals who contributed to the success of this noble and historic endeavor;
> 3. Calls this unprecedented achievement in the history of public health to the attention of all nations, which by their collective action have freed mankind of this ancient scourge and, in so doing, have demonstrated how nations working together in a common cause may further human progress.[44]

Chapter 4

Cholera

In the nineteenth century, cholera, a new, extremely frightful pandemical disease occupied the stage. The fact that scientists came to understand its causes and devise strategies for mitigating its attacks marks a historical watershed. But the episode also shows how the Public Health Approach can suffer when its advocates rely on faulty science. This chapter tells how reformers who justly focused on conditions of urban life and on prevention as a strategy for controlling infectious diseases were discredited because they relied on a speculative theory about what caused cholera.

Cholera made its first appearance in Europe in 1829. Faster travel on rivers, roads, rails, sailing vessels, and steamships enabled cholera, a gastrointestinal bacterium, to travel in the gut of sick persons from India.[1] The severe dehydration from diarrhea and vomiting that were symptoms of the dreadful disease killed its victims, sometimes within hours. Fever and ruptured small blood vessels under the skin produced small hemorrhages that gave the sick a black and blue complexion. Thus, cholera was called the blue death.

Cholera pandemics occurred on a catastrophic scale because of rural-to-urban migration that was occurring all across Europe.

Masses of poor migrants were migrating to cities that lacked adequate housing, fresh water, and sewers.[2] Unregulated urbanization resulted in overcrowded districts and soaring rates of diseases, mainly those of the gastrointestinal and respiratory tracts. Urban residents drank the water of the rivers of their cities, which they also used as receptacles for garbage and sewage and for washing clothes. These conditions were optimal for the rapid propagation of cholera.

The 1829–1833 cholera pandemic that took place in Paris is detailed in the *Rapport sur la marche et les effets du choléra-morbus dans Paris et les communes rurales du département de la Seine: année 1832* (Report on the progress and the effects of cholera-morbus in Paris and the rural communes of the Department of Seine: year 1832).[3] It totaled 207 pages plus a 200-page scientific appendix with 69 tables, 50 maps, 1 figure (shown below), and another 35 pages of documents. One of the authors, the social scientist Louis-René Villermé, had already published influential work on the causes of mortality in Paris.[4] Villermé was a member of a commission of the Royal Academy of Medicine that the French minister of the interior had tasked with identifying ways that local Boards of Health could recognize the symptoms of cholera promptly and the "curative means" they could use to defeat "this cruel malady."

During the Paris pandemic, hundreds of public health professionals, doctors, and public servants on neighborhood committees reviewed the spread of the epidemic through the city, described how city officials managed it, and tallied the number of deaths by age and gender. Figure 4.1 is evidence of the detailed statistical work that underlay this monumental document. The members of the commission had enumerated the cases and population of each administrative division of the Department of the Seine, and computed the corresponding mortality statistics. The table in the lower right of figure 4.1 lists the number of cholera deaths per 1,000 inhabitants by geographical regions (i.e., west, north, east, and south) and by administrative divisions of Paris. The "Observations" section on the lower left provides information about the design of the map. For example, the external dashed line delimits the Department of the Seine, and the solid line the City of Paris. The numbers in the central column of each region indicate the number of cholera deaths per 1,000 inhabitants for each of the corresponding communes and neighborhoods.

Cholera swept through Paris like wildfire in 1832. On February 13, a rumor spread that a porter had died in its sixth arrondissement. This was the index case. The epidemic began on March 26, when four persons died. On the next day, six more died. By April 2, the number of deaths sometimes surpassed 200 per day. The progression of the disease was frightening. By April 15, eighteen days after the epidemic began, about "12 to 13,000 were sick and 7,000 were dead." More than half of those who were infected died, often within hours. At its peak, the initial phase of the outbreak, up to June 15, killed 700 to 800 every day.[5]

Local authorities believed that miasmas were causing the disease. To eliminate the sources of miasmas, Mr. Gisquet, the prefect of police, ordered citizens to repair leaking cesspools, dry up ponds, close or cobble infected alleys, and neutralize the stench emanating from cesspools that could not be repaired. The city sprinkled the gutters of boulevards, the street pavement, and the market pavements with chlorinated water several times a day. It also increased the number of water pumps residents used for water for drinking and other household needs. Engineers redirected the waters of the Saint-Martin canal so they would wash away the mud and refuse of the ditches of Louviers Island. Although these interventions were

FIGURE 4.1. (*overleaf*) Map of subdivision of rural counties and neighborhoods of the city of Paris used for data collection, interpretation and analysis in the 1832 cholera epidemic. M. Benoiston de Chateauneuf, *Commission instituée pour recueillir les faits relatifs à l'invasion et aux effets du choléra-morbus dans le département de la Seine, 1832* (Paris: Imprimerie Royale, 1834).

DEPARTEMENT DE LA SEINE.

Classement méthodique
des 80 Communes rurales
des Arrondis. de S.t Denis et de Sceaux
et des 48 Quartiers
DE LA VILLE DE PARIS,
d'après leur situation
par rapport à la direction des Vents.

(*Voir pour les détails de Population et de Superficie le tableau précédent N.º 68*).

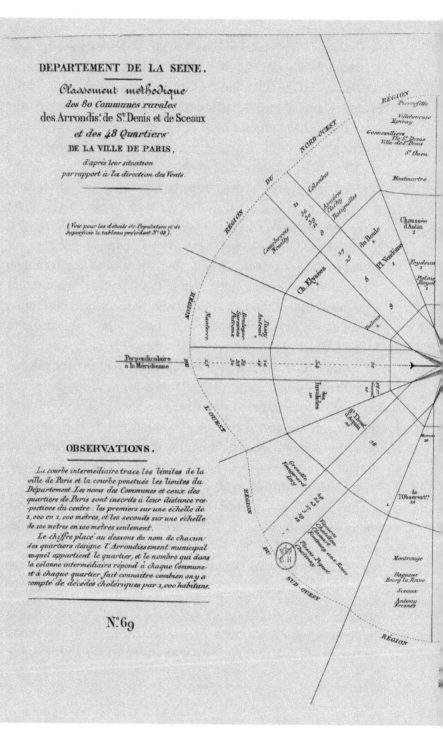

OBSERVATIONS.

La courbe intermédiaire trace les limites de la ville de Paris et la courbe ponctuée les limites du Département. Les noms des Communes et ceux des quartiers de Paris sont inscrits à leur distance respectives du centre : les premiers sur une échelle de 1,000 en 1,000 mètres, et les seconds sur une échelle de 100 mètres en 100 mètres seulement.

Le chiffre placé au dessous du nom de chacun des quartiers désigne l'Arrondissement municipal auquel appartient le quartier, et le nombre qui dans la colonne intermédiaire répond à chaque Commune et à chaque quartier fait connaître combien on y a compté de décédés cholériques par 1,000 habitans.

N.º 69

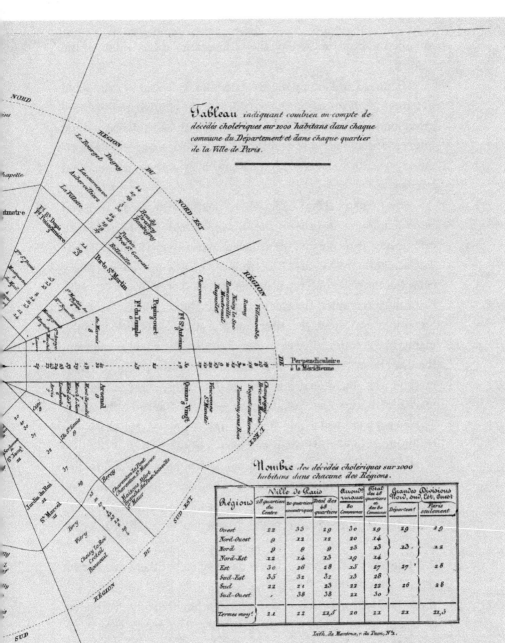

Tableau *indiquant combien on compte de décédés cholériques sur 1000 habitans dans chaque commune du Département et dans chaque quartier de la Ville de Paris.*

NORD

RÉGION DU NORD-EST

RÉGION DE L'EST

Perpendiculaire à la Méridienne

RÉGION DU SUD-EST

SUD

Nombre *des décédés cholériques sur 1000 habitans dans chacune des Régions.*

Régions	Ville de Paris			Arrond.ᵗ banlieue 80 Communes	Total des 48 quartiers et des 80 Communes	Grandes Divisions Nord, Sud, Est, Ouest	
	28 quartiers du Centre	20 quartiers excentriques	Total des 48 quartiers			Départem.ᵗ	Paris seulement
Ouest	22	33	29	30	29	29	29
Nord-Ouest	9	12	12	20	14	13	22
Nord	9	9	9	13	13		22
Nord-Est	12	14	13	19	14		
Est	30	26	28	18	27	27	28
Sud-Est	35	32	32	13	28		
Sud	22	21	23	22	22	16	28
Sud-Ouest	.	38	38	22	30		
Termes moy.s	21	22	22,5	20	22	21	22,5

Lith. de Mantoux, r. du Paon, N.4.

intended to sanitize the city, they contaminated the waters of the Seine.[6]

Home aid and ambulances carried the poor who were afflicted to temporary hospitals at the outskirts of the city, where they were given food and warm clothes. Prison authorities whitewashed the interior walls of prisons, ventilated dormitories, and used chlorinated water to wash cooking pots and beds and clean floors and latrines.

The Registre d'état civil, where deaths were recorded hired more employees to process the unusually high number of death certificates. Transporting the cadavers to cemeteries and public pits was a nightmare. At first, the minister of war provided artillery vans, but the noise of scrap iron that this kind of car was made with painfully interrupted the sleep of the inhabitants. These cars had no springs and shock absorbers and the strong jolts dislodged the planks of the coffins they were carrying, allowing a foul liquid from the dead bodies to leak into the cars and onto the pavement. This method was abandoned the next day. The army vehicles were replaced with cars that upholsterers used to transport furniture. These cars were wider and had springs. They did not shake the coffins and could carry many coffins at a time.[7]

Cadavers that piled up in homes and in hospitals and bodies were laid on the ground. They had to be buried quickly, but cemetery workers refused to work. The desolation and dread were boundless. The inhabitants of Paris, believing themselves doomed, fled the city.[8]

The outbreak began to recede on April 11, but there was a small second wave in July. The cholera epidemic in Paris lasted twenty-seven weeks, from March 26 to September 30. About 20,000 people of a population of 650,000 died, or 3.1%. The reason cholera affected the neighborhoods along the banks of the Seine is that it was the city's major source of potable water but was contaminated.[9]

Sanitary Reform

Scenarios like that in Paris occurred when cholera reached over-crowded neighborhoods with unhygienic conditions. The pandemic acutely exacerbated a situation that members of a new public health movement in France, Britain, and the United States wanted to correct by promoting urban sanitary reforms.

Urban life had different consequences for the rich and the poor. The rich enjoyed better nutrition, better hygiene, and clean water, while the new urban poor lived in overcrowded houses that had inadequate and filthy outhouses. They had poor diets, and most of the water they had access to for drinking and washing was unsanitary. The primary aim of sanitary reforms was to reduce filth and provide access to clean water. In most cities, sanitary reformers urged officials to build sewers and provide clean drinking water and encouraged homeowners to install water closets with flushable toilets. In other cities, such as Munich, the agenda of sanitary reformers also included improving ventilation and lighting in homes, greening cities, promoting better nutrition, and encouraging city officials to provide vaccines for smallpox.[10]

Sanitary reforms seemed to work. Sanitary reformers were under the impression that eliminating filth—the alleged source of miasmas—was instrumental in fighting most of the infectious diseases that plagued burgeoning metropoles. In the United Kingdom, reformers had access to data that enabled them to assess the impact of sanitary reforms on the trends in the overall number of deaths and in specific causes of death. In 1837, the bills of mortality were replaced by the compulsory registration of deaths and causes of death on a national basis. These death records included sociodemographic information. Analysis of these records revealed and/or documented differences in mortality rates between occupational groups, between residents of urban and rural districts, and between residents of small towns, middling towns, and great cities. The data showed that the excess mortality among poor populations had been slashed after 1850.[11] While it was true that the death rates for these populations decreased, it was not for the reasons sanitary reformers thought.

The Belief That Miasmas Caused Disease

In 1850, the dominant theory among sanitary reformers was that fevers were spread by foul, bad-smelling air. The concept that diseases could spread from person to person was not yet well known or accepted. The sources of foul-smelling air, such as putrefied dead animals, human excrement, and uncollected garbage, were more common in poor neighborhoods. Sanitary reformers believed that if these materials could be removed from neighborhoods, the causes of diseases would be eliminated.

Investigating the causes of diseases allegedly caused by miasmas was methodologically challenging. Even during outbreaks, fevers affected a relatively small proportion of the population even though the suspected causes (e.g., air pollution or polluted drinking water) were ubiquitous. Physicians who treated many sick patients could not identify the associations between cause and effect. The correlations between mortality rates and socioeconomic characteristics that sanitary reformers relied on also couldn't identify associations between bad air and illness. They needed to explain why everyone who was exposed to the same stench did not become sick.

To make the facts fit their beliefs, sanitary reformers relied on a theory of individual predispositions. They believed that among people similarly exposed to miasmas, susceptible people would become symptomatic and would eventually die and that people who were not predisposed would not become sick. Individual predisposition to illness caused by miasmas could stem from behavior (e.g., drinking alcohol), a person's physical morphology (e.g., weight or height) or other traits (e.g., having blond or red hair), or a person's psychology (e.g., a choleric temperament), to mention just a few of the factors sanitary reformers considered to be vulnerabilities. According to the theory of individual susceptibility, every case of cholera was caused by the combination of a miasma and idiosyncratic predispositions. Thus, the premise of the miasma hypothesis was correct in one respect: it held that some cause acted at the population level and had to be prevented by collective interventions. However, the individual susceptibility part of the theory made it untestable in population studies; it made no sense to compare a group of sick persons in which each person had contracted a form of fever for different reasons with a group of people who appeared resistant to miasmas, also each person for a different reason. The Public Health Approach of sanitary reformers was a population-based strategy that relied on an untested theory about the cause of diseases.

Sanitary reformers were satisfied with what they perceived to be the impact of social reforms on mortality trends. For example, public health in Munich, one of the most disease-ridden cities in Germany, improved rapidly under the guidance of the most influential of the reformers, Max von Pettenkofer (1818–1901).[12] Pettenkofer pioneered the establishment of scientific foundations for hygiene, which drew their roots from physiology, chemistry, and medical economics, and which he applied to clothing, bedding, dwelling, air, food, ventilation, heating, lighting, building places, soils, and their relation to air and water. One piece of evidence was the city's infant mortality rate, which had been increasing since 1825. By 1860, it had begun to decline.[13] In 1865, the University of Munich founded a first chair in hygiene for von Pettenkofer.

The Science-Based Theory of Contagion

Sanitary reforms appeared to reduce the burden of fevers (which in the nineteenth century referred to many diseases) throughout all social classes, but they did not work against cholera.

Throughout most of the nineteenth century, it remained unclear whether cholera was spread by contagion or had environmental causes linked to urban filth.[14] On July 30, 1850, about two hundred laboratory scientists and public health practitioners met in London during a cholera pandemic. The members of the London Epidemiological Society, as this group would become known, had a common interest in controlling cholera. In contrast to medical societies, they studied health and diseases "not so much in detail as in the aggregate."[15] In other words, the new society focused on population health and had two main objectives: to investigate the factors that cause or prevent diseases and to develop effective public health measures to prevent those diseases. Linking population-based research to public health policy was an important breakthrough for the Public Health Approach.

The members of the London Epidemiological Society wanted to know whether the theory that cholera was caused by miasmas was correct.[16] Evidence in favor of this theory came from authoritative sources. The previous year, William Farr (1807–1883), who worked at the Registrar General Office, had published a striking graph that showed that the mortality from cholera was higher at sea level than it was in localities at higher altitudes.[17] Sanitary reformers had postulated that heavy miasmas tended to stay low to the ground. Based on this theory, they believed that cleaning and sanitizing streets to counteract miasmas was the appropriate response to epidemics, since these actions supposedly eliminated the sources of miasmas. However, as critics of this theory had shown, the explanation for the lower rates at higher altitudes was related to population density. Large cities at higher altitudes also had high cholera mortality rates, a fact that contradicted the miasma theory.[18] But the miasma theory persisted. For example, even though a large investigation of the British General Board of Health into the causes of the cholera epidemic of 1854 in London included microscopic and chemical analyses of air in cholera wards, of water samples, and of sewage and fecal samples, the board members concluded that miasmas were the source of cholera.[19]

A minority of medical observers in the London Epidemiological Society believed that cholera was an infectious disease transmitted by a contagious agent when it was present in water, food, or the bed linen of people who had the disease. Since the mid-1820s there had been concerns that the water in London, especially the polluted Thames, was linked to illness. But at the time, the theory of contagion was difficult for most people to accept because it required a belief in the existence of small organisms that had not yet been identified. It was not until new microscopes with powerful lenses revealed minute creatures in, for example, drops of river water, that the theory of contagion developed some traction.[20]

Even though these organisms had not been identified as causal agents in the 1850s, proponents of the contagion theory, such as Dr. John Snow (1813–1858), assumed that they existed. Snow devised population studies that were consistent with the theory that microorganisms caused cholera. The contagion theory lent itself well to comparisons of groups of people who had been exposed to contaminated food, water, or bed linen with groups that had not been in contact with these things. Still, contagionists were challenged to test their theory because stench was always present where there was cholera. Sanitary reformers continued to argue that cholera was caused by an agent in the air people breathed. The only way to conclusively prove the validity of the contagion theory was to design a research strategy that separated the effects of polluted water from those of air pollution. That is what John Snow did in 1854.[21] Using death certificates, he was able to show that among London residents who lived in the same house blocks and thus breathed the same air, a larger proportion died from cholera when they drank cholera-polluted water that had been pumped from the Thames to the center of London than their neighbors who drank clean water that was transported to London from the countryside.[22]

However, Snow's population-based epidemiological study attracted little attention when it was published.[23]

The Natural Experiment

Whether cholera was a contagious disease or was spread by miasmas had policy implications. If cholera was a contagious disease that spread from person to person, then preventing contagion required isolating sick people, quarantining ships and migrating populations, and closing markets. These means of prevention, however, paralyzed the businesses of merchants and shopkeepers with limited benefit. Quarantining ships and imported merchandise, isolating individuals, and creating cordons sanitaires did not seem to prevent the spread of cholera. Moreover, from the perspective of sanitary reformers, the policy responses the contagion theory implied did not remove the filth from the neighborhoods of the workforce the economy needed. In their view, if cholera was spread by miasmas, then local markets, fairs, and other places where people gathered could remain open, and business could go on as usual as long as they were cleaned and sanitized.

Because sanitary reformers relied on the speculative theory that miasmas were the means by which cholera was spread, they failed to protect populations from the recurring waves of cholera and may even have contributed to wider spread of the disease. Washing street refuse and the contents of cesspools from districts experiencing an outbreak of cholera into rivers contaminated a main source of drinking water for urban residents. Contaminated water then disseminated an outbreak that might have remained local or might have disseminated more slowly to the rest of the city.

That is what happened when a cholera epidemic reached the German cities of Hamburg and Altona in 1892.[24] The two cities were part of one urban area that had different political administrations. Both drew their drinking water from the Elbe River. Altona officials, who subscribed to contagionist principles, used a system that filtered river water through gravel to remove its bacterial contents before sending it to faucets. In Hamburg, where officials followed the recommendations of sanitary reformers, river water was not seen as a source of miasmas and was therefore sent unfiltered to water faucets throughout the city. When a cholera epidemic hit Hamburg and Altona in 1892, Hamburg lost 8,616 residents to the disease (1.34% of the city's population). This was a very high mortality rate; as a point of comparison, in London, mortality rates from cholera never exceeded 0.66%.[25] In contrast, only 328 people died from cholera in Altona (0.2% of the population). When officials saw these numbers, the pro-contagion administration took control of Hamburg and imposed case isolation and quarantine until the outbreak receded.

The 1892 cholera epidemic in Hamburg symbolized the defeat of the ideas of sanitary reformers, more so than any studies the contagionists, such as John Snow, had published. It provided a convincing demonstration of the dangerousness of the miasma theory. The disastrous outbreak in Hamburg discredited the belief in miasmas.[26]

In historian Richard J. Evans's analysis,

The resulting cholera epidemic of 1892 exposed [Hamburg] to the condemnation of world opinion. Like all epidemics, it was not an autonomous, chance occurrence beyond the reach of human power: cholera, more than most diseases, indeed, was the product of human agency, of social inequality and political unrest, of industry and empire. It came at a time when economic and social inequalities in the city had reached unprecedented dimensions.[27]

Evans's analysis suggests that the commitment of most sanitary reformers to social equality was weak. Inequality in Hamburg had not improved since 1850. Many of the movement's members were less concerned about the welfare of the poor than they were about how endemic and epidemic disease caused by defective sewers or infected food affected the entire community, which of course included the wealthy elite.[28] Historian Christopher Hamlin has noted that British sanitarians focused on filth and neglected work, wages, and food.[29] As George Rosen notes, sanitary reformers were primarily promoting economic and political liberalism, not socialism.[30]

Science-Based Public Health

The sanitary reform movement illustrates the risks of not relying on science-based data in the field of public health. The sanitary reformers of the nineteenth century got halfway there: they understood the population dimension of health. In an unprecedented urbanistic effort, they helped Western societies control the unhygienic living conditions that accompanied the massive rural-to-urban migration, industrialization, and urbanization. They helped shape modern urban life so that it could provide the healthy working class the economy needed while mitigating the extreme class antagonisms of that period. As Amy Fairchild and colleagues note:

> New housing was now required to have indoor plumbing and connections to water and sewer lines, which were replacing wells and privies. Tenement laws mandated that all rooms in newly constructed buildings have windows that opened to the outside. Restrictions on housing density and new nuisance laws began to have an effect on rates of tuberculosis and other diseases. Laws governing foodstuffs, meat, and milk as well as regulation of "noxious trades" such as slaughterhouses and tanneries began to produce improvements in health. In rural areas, malaria, yellow fever, and pellagra were addressed through engineering and social reforms from the draining of swamps to the provision of better diets and work to poor sharecroppers both Black and White.[31]

Sanitary reformers documented the trends in population size, births, deaths, and life expectancy with detailed statistical tables and graphs.[32] However, their legacy was tarnished by their reliance on a speculative theory that related disease to air that had been polluted by putrefied organic matter.

They correctly believed that improving drainage, cleaning streets and houses, and removing garbage required civil engineering, not medicine.[33] This reasoning appeared to be supported by statistics that showed that between cholera pandemics, all health indicators were improving for society as a whole. Yet this thinking had a fundamental flaw: clean air was not more important than clean water, uncontaminated food, and strategies that reduced the spread of contagious diseases. The catastrophic epidemic of cholera in Hamburg 1892 harmed the legacy of the sanitarians. In the eyes of the public, the magnitude of their long-term achievements diminished.[34]

The Germ Theory of Disease

For some portions of some populations, the hygiene of daily life in 1900 was very different from that of 1800. The societies that were healthier in 1900 than they had been in 1850 appeared to have been saved by the progress of the field of bacteriology. The scientists who believed in contagion tested their theory in populations. Lab-based science became the image of public health instead of one of its subfields. The field of bacteriology became much more reliable and accurate, and bacteriology labs became the source of new knowledge that shaped public health policies and recommendations.[35] Labs identified microorganisms and urged public officials to isolate the sick. The debate about whether diseases were caused by miasmas or germs was over, and doctors and public health officials were largely converted to the germ theory of disease. Instead of controlling people's environment, as sanitarians had done, public health officials turned to controlling specific communicable diseases. With the advent of antibiotics in the twentieth century, public health increasingly became an offshoot of medical care.

Bacteriologists identified microscopic agents that caused most of the prevalent diseases of the early twentieth century. They associated cholera, tuberculosis, puerperal fever, bacterial pneumonia, scarlet fever, typhoid fever, plague, and diphtheria with specific bacterial microorganisms. The causes of other diseases such as measles and the flu were not known until viral disease agents were discovered in the 1920s. Bacteriologists developed specific protective treatments against anthrax and rabies, preventive treatments against typhoid, and curative serums for diphtheria and tetanus using the specific bacteria associated with these infections. They inspired surgeons to practice disinfection; at first only for their instruments but later for the entire surgical environment. This greatly reduced mortality from septicemia.[36]

These were tremendously important achievements, but as repeatedly emphasized by public health historian Anne Hardy, the contribution of bacteriology was overestimated. The germ-focused approach of bacteriology was easy to understand: preventing the dissemination of germs that caused diseases made sense. However, it was not true that focusing on the germ was sufficient to prevent outbreaks and control the propagation of the disease.[37] First, laboratory facilities capable of responding in real time to an outbreak were rare until well into the twentieth century, although there were some exceptions to this generalization. (For example, lab facilities were crucial for stemming epidemic meningitis outbreaks among British troops during World War I.) Second, laboratory methods were useless when an epidemic was transmitted via an unusual route that had not been established using epidemiologic methods. Investigation of outbreaks of unknown origin was needed to discover that cow's milk could transmit tuberculosis, oysters could transmit typhoid,[38] or powdered milk for infant feeding could cause fatal diarrhea.[39] Once this background work was done, lab scientists knew where to search for the germs.

A Missed Opportunity

The London Epidemiological Society explicitly linked research and public health. Unfortunately, its reliance on an obsolete theory became a liability for its members. Sanitary reformers clearly understood the difference between medicine and the population approach to fighting disease. Yet their belief in individual susceptibility to miasmas had devastating implications for the many people who died in cities that followed their policy recommendations.

It is reasonable to think that had sanitary reformers paid more attention to the scientific background of the miasma theory that guided their actions, the role of preventive public health could have been very different in the following century. Professionals and academics such as Rudolf Virchow (1821–1902) in Berlin, Max von Pettenkofer in Munich, and William Farr in London, all sanitary reformers, were among the most respected scientific personalities of the nineteenth century. Had sanitary reformers designed comparative studies like that of John Snow, they could have avoided the Hamburg disaster in 1892, and their role in the twentieth century might not have been discredited. The sanitary reformers' vision of public health would have benefited tremendously from integrating bacteriology instead of competing with it. It is conceivable that a domain of government activity dedicated to population thinking about public health would have been developed to a much greater extent in the nineteenth and early twentieth centuries and would have been independent of the individual approach to health that characterized the medical field.

Chapter 5

Tuberculosis

Tuberculosis became a dominant concern at the turn of the twentieth century. Pulmonary tuberculosis is an airborne bacterial disease that began affecting human populations at some point after humans began farming cattle. The spontaneous evolution of the disease is characterized by a slow onset. It begins with great fatigue, then the patient begins experiencing fever in the evening. Eventually the patient coughs up blood and loses weight. Before treatments were developed for this disease, patients would die after months or years of sickness. In the nineteenth century, tuberculosis was called consumption, as it caused patients to waste away. Until the mid-twentieth century, it affected almost every family in the West, killed many in the same family, and produced countless orphans. The bacterium that causes tuberculosis was invisible, and because symptoms did not appear immediately after exposure, the cause was not established until 1882, when Robert Koch (1843–1910) described the tubercle bacillus.

The mortality rate from tuberculosis can be tracked in the United Kingdom from the seventeenth century. It may have declined in the eighteenth century but came back brutally among the newly urbanized populations of the nineteenth century who lived in overcrowded conditions and were poorly fed. In the late nineteenth and early twentieth centuries, tuberculous patients were isolated when possible in rural, mountainous, and cold areas. To reduce transmission, spitting in public places became prohibited in several parts of the United States.[1] In 1921, a vaccine was developed from an attenuated form of the bacillus that was 50% effective.[2] Better nutrition, which reduces the risk of acquiring tuberculosis or of dying from it, and better hygiene—for example, segregating those infected with respiratory tuberculosis and milk pasteurization against bovine tuberculosis—resulted in the decline of the disease throughout the twentieth century.

Tuberculosis was difficult to study. Unlike other infectious diseases, it did not have a clear-cut onset. Moreover, there was no clear means of tracking the transmission from person to person. Years could pass between the exposure to a contagious, tuberculous person and the appearance of symptoms in the contaminated person. The infection could last for decades and its clinical symptoms could recur. After the discovery of the tubercle bacillus and the rejection of the miasma theory, some people believed that the disease affected only people who had a hereditary predisposition because it seemed to run in families. Determining its social causes and finding an effective treatment required the rigorous implementation of the two main methodologies of group comparison: the cohort study and the randomized controlled trial.

Challenging Eugenics

In the early twentieth century, public health advocates were obsessed with the idea that tuberculosis posed an existential threat to the human species. They were fascinated by the concept of combining the germ theory of disease with the Darwinian theory of natural selection, a major scientific insight of the nineteenth century. Combining bacteriology with the idea that the concept of survival of the fittest could be applied to human populations became known as eugenics: a theory positing that it was possible and desirable to increase the occurrence of heritable characteristics within a human population that would allegedly improve the human race. Eugenics took two forms: negative eugenics discouraged or prevented the reproduction of allegedly genetically inferior individuals and populations, and positive eugenics encouraged the reproduction of allegedly genetically superior individuals and populations. The theory of eugenics was developed by Francis Galton, Charles Darwin's half-cousin. Darwin did not embrace the views of more fervent eugenicists, including his pro-eugenics son Leonard Darwin, and was very careful about applying the concept of natural selection to human populations.

Eugenics ideas were widespread in the United States in the early decades of the twentieth century.[3] In the period 1907 to 1926, twenty-three US states enacted legislation that provided for some form of eugenic sterilization. Between 1907 and 1925, 6,244 people had been surgically sterilized in these states.[4] These early sterilization programs targeted white men and women suffering from some form of physical or mental "defect," but later in the twentieth century women and people of color increasingly became the target.[5] One of the most popular expressions of positive eugenics in rural America was the Better Babies Contest, an annual event at state fairs that brought public health and animal breeding together in a unique way.[6]

Eugenics was a speculative theory that combined a population perspective and Darwinian natural selection with a concept of individual, genetic susceptibility that was difficult to identify. Bacteriologists had established that the tubercle bacillus was the bacterium that caused tuberculosis. They had proved that the bacillus was always present in infected animals, never present in healthy animals, and could transmit tuberculosis when it was injected into a healthy animal. Eugenicists believed that another factor contributed to the cause of the disease: people who developed tuberculosis when they were exposed to the tubercle bacillus had a genetic susceptibility that would have been eliminated by Darwinian natural selection but was artificially kept prevalent by modern medicine and sanatoria.

Eugenics advocates argued that under primitive conditions of natural selection, people who carried the gene that made them susceptible to tuberculosis would have been eliminated but that improvements in medical care and the growth of insurance and social benefits during the late nineteenth century had artificially allowed tuberculous people to survive, reproduce, and taint the genetic makeup of humans. Simple observations seemed to support this theory. In 1800, tuberculous patients died because of severe protein-calorie malnutrition, pulmonary hemorrhage, and fever. They were consumed by the disease. By 1900, middle-class tuberculous patients had nutritious diets and were often isolated for a period in specialized centers called sanatoria. Tuberculous people could survive, live apparently normal lives, and have families. It had become a very common disease.

Eugenicist ideas about tuberculosis were not tested empirically until the early twentieth century, in part because it was not possible to identify who was genetically susceptible from the rest of the population. In Stuttgart, Dr. Wilhelm Weinberg (1862–1937), a physician of general medicine and obstetrics and an outstanding scientist, found a creative way to test the validity of eugenics theories. He speculated that children born to parents who had died from tuberculosis were likely to carry a susceptibility factor that predisposed them to contract the disease. In 1910, he became the chair of the Stuttgart Society for Racial Hygiene. (In Germany, racial hygiene was the term for eugenics in the early decades of the twentieth century.)

Weinberg wanted to establish whether inherited tuberculosis conferred a survival advantage that would progressively come to dominate the "well-born" and therefore weaken the genetic quality of the human species. Weinberg defined as genetically susceptible to become tuberculous a person who had lost a parent to tuberculosis. By identifying a proxy for genetic susceptibility (the loss of a parent to the disease), Weinberg made possible a shift to a population perspective on the eugenics theory of tuberculosis transmission.

In *The Children of the Tuberculous*, published in 1913, Weinberg described the methods and results of a study that followed 25,786 children from birth to age 20 who had been born to 7,098 parents living in Stuttgart. The study compared retrospectively, using registry data, the mortality of children whose parents had died of tuberculosis with that of children whose parents had died from other causes. Weinberg found that the life expectancy of children whose father or mother had died of tuberculosis was shorter than those whose father or mother had died of other causes. Children whose father had died of tuberculosis had a nearly 47% chance of dying before age 20. If the mother died of the disease, the likelihood that her children would die before age 20 was 48%. In contrast, children whose father or mother died of other causes had a lower, 40% chance of dying before age 20.[7]

This design is now referred to as a cohort study, a study that follows two (or more) groups of people across time. Since the children of the tuberculous parents lived a shorter life than those of the nontuberculous parents, the racial hygienic theory according to which susceptibility to tuberculosis was becoming more common was debunked: the survival advantage was on the side of the children who did not have tuberculous parents. However, there was a social gradient: children in the upper social classes lived substantially longer on average than those in lower social classes. Weinberg's science-based results had a reasonable public health implication: the impact of tuberculosis could be mitigated by improving the living conditions of the poor.

There is no indication that Weinberg's book had any impact on the decline of eugenics. The theory lost its popularity in the 1930s and 1940s because it lacked scientific foundations and because the

Nazis used it to justify their sterilization and euthanization of allegedly defective Germans and their race-based extermination of Jews and other populations in concentration camps.[8]

Popularizing the Concept of Fair Comparisons

After World War I, statisticians began to favor the concept of a randomized trial that included a control group and a treatment group. Many doctors were opposed to this methodology. They interpreted it as preventing some patients from receiving treatment for the sake of scientific research. This issue was the theme of Sinclair Lewis's 1925 novel *Arrowsmith*, which director John Ford treated in a film of the same title in 1931. The book and the movie depict the clash between researchers who sought a population approach as a way to prevent epidemics from devastating societies and clinicians who were focused on their responsibility to individual patients.

Lewis may have chosen to feature an outbreak of plague in his novel because the world had been threatened by an epidemic of pneumonic plague in Manchuria in 1911 that had killed an estimated 60,000 people. *Yersinia pestis* had only to cross the Pacific Ocean to reach California. Although the outbreak did not reach the United States, fears were high that it would do so in 1911.[9] Pneumonic plague is so contagious and so deadly that its victims tend to die close to where they are infected. As a result, the 1911 epidemic remained local.

In the novel, an epidemic of plague was raging in the West Indies. The populations of the Caribbean islands affected by the outbreak were terrified. Dr. Martin Arrowsmith believed he had an antidote and wanted to test it by giving it only to half the island first. If it worked to protect that group, he would give it to the other half too.

The novel and the movie described the relatively new concept of the randomized trial: comparing groups that are identical on every aspect, and only differ because one receives a therapeutic or preventive intervention and the other not. The technical term is "randomization," from random or chance, since the intervention could be allocated by tossing a coin, and the study design is the "randomized controlled trial," as one group serves as control for the other.

When Martin Arrowsmith declares his intention of conducting a randomized controlled trial to test the effectiveness of his antidote, the governor of the West Indies, Sir Robert, and the doctors on the board of health of the island of St. Hubert are outraged. They only see a lack of humanity. Sir Robert interprets the project as an attempt to use the inhabitants of the island as guinea pigs and refuses to facilitate the project. One doctor tells Arrowsmith that he calls himself a doctor but wants to see half his patients die.

In the novel, one man offers to run the trial in a remote indigenous community on a neighboring island that was affected by the epidemic. The population was divided into two equal parts. One of them was injected with Dr. Arrowsmith's serum, the other half was not. The untreated half of the parish was much more heavily affected than those who had been treated. A case or two occurred among those who had received the serum, but among the others there were dozens of victims. The serum was proved to be effective. Both Lewis's novel and Ford's film treatment introduced the concept of a fair group comparison to the public.

The 1947 Streptomycin Trial

In 1947, the method of comparing groups of patients to assess the efficacy of an intervention, the randomized controlled trial, was used to assess the efficacy of streptomycin. Before 1945, the efficacy of new therapies in medical science was rarely tested. In the case of most new treatments, it was not known whether they would be effective and prescribing them could have dangerous effects.

Assessing the efficacy and side effects of medical treatments could only be done at a group level. Randomization was the new idea: if the intervention modified the course of the disease in the treated group but not in the control group, the observed difference could be attributed to the treatment. A simple form of randomization is to assign study participants to the two groups by tossing a coin. For example, if the coin lands on heads, the study participant is assigned to the treatment group. If the coin lands on tails, the study participant is assigned to the control group. The order of the tails and heads is unpredictable, resulting in two groups comprising participants selected haphazardly, and therefore comparable. Many randomizing techniques are more reliable than tossing a coin, but the principle is the same: important determinants of the outcome of the intervention, such as age and gender, will tend to be equally represented in both randomized groups.

In 1943, laboratory experiments in tuberculous guinea pigs showed that streptomycin, an antibiotic produced by a fungus, was toxic to the bacterium that caused tuberculosis. However, the newly created British National Health Service felt that the new drug was very expensive. That is why the British Medical Research Council tested it on humans to see whether it was effective in clinical practice.

Tuberculous patients were randomized into two groups. The treatment group received streptomycin and the control group was treated only with bed rest.[10] This randomized controlled trial used sound techniques for allocating the treatment and concealing from the doctors in charge of the patients included in the study the sequence in which streptomycin or bed rest were allocated. Two grams per day of streptomycin were given intramuscularly to the treatment group at six-hour intervals. During the first six months of the trial, only four people died among fifty-five patients (7.3%) in the treatment group, compared to fourteen deaths among fifty-two patients (27%) in the control group. The streptomycin experiment showed how population thinking enriched clinical medicine (i.e., individually prescribed treatments). Physicians began increasingly incorporating the results of randomized controlled trials in their clinical practice.[11]

Streptomycin and isoniazid, another wonder drug, further reduced the already declining mortality rate from tuberculosis, which has continued to remain low. However, the disease can thrive in places where malnutrition is prevalent, cases cannot be isolated, and immune-suppressing diseases are present. In 2020, 10 million people were infected with tuberculosis, and 1.5 million people died from it worldwide.[12] African regions with a high prevalence of HIV/AIDS are greatly affected. Ending the tuberculosis epidemic by 2030 is among the health targets of the United Nations Sustainable Development Goals.

Progress in the Public Health Approach

The methodological sophistication required to analyze endemic diseases created pressure to train personnel in the newly developing statistical approaches that were emerging in England. In 1903, Karl Pearson's Biometric Laboratory (later the Galton Laboratory for National Eugenics) at University College London developed increasingly sophisticated mathematical methods for conducting research such as correlations and statistical tests.

There was also a need for personnel that had expertise in toxicology, hygiene, and bacteriology. Staff of the Rockefeller Sanitary Commission for the Eradication of Hookworm Disease had difficulty finding public health professionals in US South who had the background for the work the commission was doing. The context called for a new profession. In 1912, Tulane University, in New Orleans, established a school of hygiene and tropical medicine, including public health. In 1913, the Harvard-MIT School of Health Officers was founded, to provide training for public health professionals. In 1916, the Rockefeller Foundation funded the Johns Hopkins School of Hygiene and Public Health, which opened its doors on October 1, 1918, at the height of the great influenza pandemic. It also funded the

London School of Hygiene & Tropical Medicine, which opened in 1924. The DeLamar Institute of Public Health at Columbia University opened in 1922.[13]

In 1927, the London School of Hygiene & Tropical Medicine appointed William Whiteman Carlton Topley (1886–1944) to the chair in bacteriology and immunology and epidemiologist and statistician Major Greenwood (1880–1949) as the first professor of epidemiology and vital statistics.[14] These appointments formalized the teaching of public health in London. The school also offered advanced courses for students specializing in epidemiology. Because of Britain's obligations to its colonies, the study of tropical medicine and hygiene formed a significant part of the curriculum. The school also trained students aiming for careers as local medical officers of health or school medical officers. Teaching and research at the school featured topics such as Bacillus Calmette-Guérin vaccines for tuberculosis and measles prophylaxis.

These developments provided the foundations for a science-based dimension of the Public Health Approach that had been missing in the sanitary reform movement. The approach began to be applied to a wider range of health determinants than infectious diseases in the first decade of the twentieth century. However, the four years of World War I interrupted the progress of the development of science-based public health. The Great Influenza, a furiously fatal epidemic, peaked in the autumn of 1918. There followed a decade of slow economic recovery, a worldwide economic recession during the Great Depression, and six more years of all-out war during World War II. The 30 years of quasi-permanent world chaos may have masked the depth and speed at which the epidemiological profile of Western societies was changing. While mortality rates from infectious disease were decreasing, the death rates from cancer and heart diseases were increasing. The frequency of these diseases, which were already on the rise during the interwar period, increased dramatically after World War II.

Chapter 6

Cancer and Cardiovascular Diseases

The acquisition of population survey data, which was new in the twentieth century, provided information that pointed toward some of the causes of the epidemics of cancer and cardiovascular diseases and brought them to the attention of the broad public.[1] Surveys collected data about behavior and morbidity that census data and death certificates did not adequately provide.[2]

As the burden of infectious diseases such as tuberculosis and typhoid or of perinatal and childhood mortality declined in Western societies, public health researchers shifted their priority from infectious diseases to focusing on lung and breast cancer, and coronary diseases.[3] The long course of these diseases, which sometimes span lifetimes, appeared to be related to potentially modifiable behavioral causes such as traumatized breast nipples (incriminated in the 1920s as a cause of breast cancer), diet, or addiction to tobacco. Therefore, the thinking went, these diseases might be preventable. However, identifying the causes was not straightforward because these diseases were still relatively rare and the length of time between the onset of the causal behavior and their onset could be long. This was a new situation for epidemiological researchers.

The shifts in perspective that occurred as researchers attempted to understand and devise recommendations for changes in behavior that would control the epidemics of lung cancer and cardiovascular diseases resulted in two major developments for the Public Health Approach: a method for assessing causality based on population data and a population strategy for modifying health-related behaviors.

Population-Based Causality

Cigarettes dispense nicotine, a highly addictive substance. After new manufacturing processes in the early twentieth century reduced the costs of producing cigarettes, markets were inundated with them, and consumption grew exponentially. During the two world wars, governments provided free tobacco to soldiers on both sides of the battlefield. Many nonsmoking soldiers in the German and Allied armies became nicotine addicts.[4]

In the 1920s, research showed that tobacco tar was carcinogenic in animals.[5] By the early 1930s it was known that smoking was associated with cancer in humans,[6] yet as late as 1945, there was no consensus about the causes of cancer. The population perspective on tobacco and cancer was still in its infancy. The common perception before World War II was that smoking was a healthy habit. It was widely believed that tobacco helped people relax and concentrate. A 1936 editorial in *Scientific American* called cigarettes "a package of rest."[7] When cigarettes were at the peak of their popularity, smoking was a "cool" practice, and movie stars considered role models, such as Marlene Dietrich or Humphrey Bogart, were often depicted with cigarettes in films. However, in 1945, reports from surveys and vital statistics in the United States and the United Kingdom indicated that both smoking habits and the burden of cancer had both increased significantly.[8] To understand the link between these two observations better, researchers designed epidemiological studies.

At first, researchers sought environmental causes for the increase in rates of cancer. The twentieth century had seen the replacement of horse-powered vehicles by cars and their combustion engines. The air stank because of the pollution from motor vehicle exhaust, industrial waste products, dust and fumes from tarred roads, and the burning of heating fuels.[9] However, it was difficult to demonstrate the links between these changes and cancer given the early stage of epidemiological methods in the mid-twentieth century.

In 1950, a series of population studies consistently reported that groups of people who suffered from lung cancer included more heavy smokers than the comparison group of people who did not have lung cancer. In 1951, two British researchers conducted a large cohort study. They sent a letter to all British doctors that asked them about their smoking habits. Over 40,000 doctors responded to the survey questions. Those who reported that they were smokers answered questions about how old they were when they started smoking, how much they smoked, and whether they smoked pipes or cigarettes. Those who reported that they were ex-smokers answered the same questions about their former smoking habits plus a question about when they stopped smoking. Twenty-nine months later, the researchers tallied the number of deaths due to lung cancer among the 789 respondees who had died: the doctors who were smokers in 1951 had a risk of developing lung cancer fourteen times higher than those who did not smoke. These results were published in a detailed article in the *British Medical Journal* in 1954.[10] These findings were confirmed by the results of a study of 180,000 members of the American Cancer Society that was published in the *Journal of the American Medical Association* that same year.[11]

In response to the fact that epidemiological studies consistently confirmed the health risks of smoking, the tobacco industry launched a disinformation campaign in the United States that saturated the media with incorrect information about the health benefits of cigarettes.[12] Some of these ads featured doctors who spoke about which brand of cigarettes they preferred. The implicit message of such ads was that smoking must be safe if doctors did it.

Some statisticians of the 1950s felt that the epidemiological studies of tobacco and cancer to date were weak in theory and design and that they did not satisfy the statistical canons of valid inference. One core principle was that all statistical studies of the same problem should provide the same answer.[13] The two groups that a study compared needed to be identical in every respect except that one group received or participated in the "treatment" related to the issue being studied. When all other variables among the two groups were identical, the effect of the exposure would stand out. These were called Fisher's standards, named for Ronald A. Fisher (1890–1962), the British statistician who had formulated them in *The Design of Experiments*, an influential text that was first published in 1935.[14] A typical question in the book was to test whether one could trust "a lady [who] declares that by tasting a cup of tea made with milk she can discriminate whether the milk or the tea infusion was first added to the cup."[15]

The epidemiological questions were of a very different nature. None of the epidemiological studies of the 1950s relating tobacco to lung cancer met Fisher's standards. None used randomization, and each study was designed differently. Some statisticians noted the inconsistent designs from such studies and highlighted their many weak spots.[16]

Despite these irregularities in study design, by the end of the 1950s, a major segment of the scientific community shared the opinion that the most reasonable interpretation of the evidence was that smoking caused lung cancer. After about ten years of intense scrutiny, support was growing for the idea that tobacco consumption played a role in the epidemic of lung cancer researchers were documenting. Both the United States Public Health Service and the British Medical Research Council issued warnings about excessive smoking in the 1950s. By 1962, the British Royal College of Physicians published a comprehensive report that examined many studies from around the world on the relationship between tobacco consumption and lung cancer.[17] The report concluded that "the strong statistical association between smoking, especially of cigarettes, and lung cancer is most simply explained on a causal basis. This is supported by compatible . . . laboratory and pathological evidence."[18]

The foundations for such statements were elusive because the principles of causality still relied on thinking based on individuals, not groups. For instance, in order to establish the cause of tuberculosis, Robert Koch had shown that any guinea pig inoculated with the tubercle bacillus would develop the disease. However, researchers knew that only 10% of the heavy smokers would develop lung cancer and that the life expectancy of only about 50% of smokers would be shortened.[19] How could cigarette smoking be established as a cause of lung cancer when only a portion of smokers got sick or died because of it?

The watershed for the switch from an individual to a population approach to causality happened in the context of studies of the relationship between tobacco and lung cancer. In 1961, the leaders of the American Cancer Society, the American Public Health Association, the American Heart Association, and the National Tuberculosis Association sent a letter to President John F. Kennedy that urged him to form a presidential commission to study "the widespread implications of the tobacco problem."[20] The letter had apparently no impact on the president. However, after having being asked at a news conference about his administration's intentions to address the piling up of scientific studies indicating that smoking was a health concern, Kennedy asked Surgeon General Luther Terry to look into the issue.[21] In 1963, Terry asked the United States Public

Health Service to assemble an Advisory Committee whose task would be to examine the effects of smoking on health and make recommendations.[22] The ten members of the committee that was assembled had been deemed trustworthy by both the US government and the tobacco industry.[23] In fact, some members were heavy smokers.[24]

The committee members noted that a causal relationship could not be inferred from a single epidemiological study that showed that cigarette smoking was associated with cancer. They turned to a system for evaluating studies of the relationship between tobacco consumption and cancer. They established a set of criteria for evaluating whether it was valid to accept that smoking caused cancer:

(a) *The consistency of the association:* The committee underlined that diverse epidemiological studies, whether they compared cases and controls or smokers with nonsmokers, found an association between cigarette smoking and lung cancer.

(b) *The strength of the association:* Committee members noted that even though not all smokers got sick, their risk of dying from lung cancer was many times greater than that of nonsmokers, and the risk increased when a person smoked 5, 10, or 20 cigarettes per day.

(c) *The specificity of the association:* Lung cancer was rare among nonsmokers.

(d) *The temporal relationship of the association:* The habit of smoking began years and sometimes decades before the cancer occurred.

(e) *The coherence of the association with "known facts in the natural history and biology of the disease"*:[25] For example, the increase in lung cancer mortality in the United States had followed an increase in per capita consumption of cigarettes.[26]

In *Ashes to Ashes: America's Hundred-Year Cigarette War, the Public Health, and the Unabashed Triumph of Philip Morris*, Richard Kluger described the moment when a subgroup of committee members that included a doctor, a statistician, and an epidemiologist, who was a heavy smoker, reached a consensus about which criteria they would use to ensure statistical rigor in their study of the relationship between tobacco consumption and disease:

> After much shooting of pool and talking shop, the little group had its final dinner together, wreathed in smoke from all their cigarettes, and at the end it was [Ruel] Stallones, a witty companion and incisive thinker, who pulled it all together. The question before them had been what criteria had to be met before medical science could conclude that the statistical case against smoking as the prime cause of lung cancer had been proven. "This is what I think we've been talking about," Stallones said and, taking an empty pack of Luckies from his pocket and tearing it apart, scrawled on the inside surface of the wrapper: "The consistency of the statistical association, the strength of the association, specificity of the association, and the coherence of the association."[27]

In 1964, at the end of thirteen months of examination of the evidence, the committee unanimously concluded that there was a causal link between tobacco and lung cancer, at least for men. Too few cases had been studied among women to draw firm conclusions.

Cigarette sales in the United States peaked in 1964 and then declined. Lung cancer mortality followed the same trajectory with an approximately twenty-year delay. We are still witnessing the significance of the achievements of the 1950s and 1960s in the declining smoking trends in Western societies. Kenneth E. Warner reviewed this legacy on the fiftieth anniversary of the US surgeon general's 1964 report.[28] Given the amount of evidence that had accrued by the mid-1950s, the link could have been deemed causal much earlier, but it took until 1964 for the issue to be settled enough for large-scale governmental action.[29]

Nonsmoking flight attendants who worked in smoke-filled cabins of airplanes for years and had developed lung cancer filed (in 1991) and won (in 1997) a class action against the producer Philip Morris. The tobacco industry agreed to pay $300 million to establish a medical foundation to study illnesses linked to tobacco smoke.[30] The recognition that passive smoking was harmful led states and localities to prohibit smoking in public places. As of January 1, 2023, 62.5% of the US population is protected from secondhand smoke exposure by local or statewide smokefree laws in nonhospitality workplaces, restaurants, and bars.[31]

Such public health attainments were achieved by an outstandingly persistent generation of public health practitioners and researchers who slowly brought the Public Health Approach to the level needed to meet the historical challenge: the recognition that causality could be based on group comparisons and epidemiological associations. This was the methodology used in the 1964 US Surgeon General's report *Smoking and Health*, which authoritatively concluded that a causal link existed between cigarette smoking and lung cancer. The Surgeon General's Advisory Committee had provided a formal procedure for establishing causation.

The criteria the Surgeon General's Advisory Committee used for inferring causality were later enriched by the British epidemiologist Austin Bradford Hill in a seminal article titled "The Environment and Disease: Association or Causation?"[32] Although many attempts have been made to generate different methods of determining an inference of causation, the criteria the Advisory Committee established have been applied almost systematically in epidemiology and public health since 1964.[33]

The causal criteria approach was based on both science and population thinking. In contrast, the argument that smoking was a hereditary trait was speculative. Criticisms of the epidemiological studies that concluded that smoking is a cause of cancer based on the argument that smokers were genetically different from non-smokers seemed to hearken back to eugenics thinking. For example, in the late 1950s, Ronald Fisher dismissed the findings of epidemiological studies because they could not rule out a genetic factor as a common cause of both smoking and cancer.[34] A genetically predisposed constitution, he argued, was what made people "take to the pipe and [not] take to cigarettes, just as there are other men who would never take to a pipe but constantly feel the need of cigarettes."[35] To support his theory, Fisher reported that identical twins showed closer similarity and fewer divergences in their smoking habits than fraternal ones.[36] Fisher's speculative argument about the genetic basis of smoking was surprising. A genetic cause could not explain the 22 percent increase in mortality from lung cancer among English men aged 25 and older from 1952 to 1961 and its reduction, during the same period, among the participants in the 1951 British study of doctors.[37] What gene could increase smoking prevalence and mortality in the general population and decrease it among doctors?

Population-Based Epidemiology

At the close of World War II, heart attacks appeared to have become increasingly widespread. They often killed middle-aged men suddenly. A first step was identifying causes. Cardiovascular diseases differed profoundly from of lung cancer. The effect of tobacco on cancer stood out because in study after study, tobacco could be the only characteristics in an individual behavior or biology that was linked to lung cancer, and nonsmokers rarely had lung cancer. In contrast, cardiovascular diseases could be caused by many things. A poor diet, obesity, high blood pressure or high cholesterol, and high

blood glucose were all potential risk factors in addition to tobacco.[38] In terms of rigorous epidemiological study, it would be
difficult to determine whether one or more of these factors acted
alone or if different combinations of these possible factors caused
heart disease.

In 1947, the United States Public Health Service launched the
Framingham Heart Study, named for Framingham, a Massachusetts town of 28,000 located 23 miles west of Boston.[39] This was a
large-scale study that focused on the causes, prevention, and treatment of cardiovascular diseases. Researchers conducted biennial
examinations of 5,200 white men and women to determine whether
cardiovascular diseases were associated with slow-acting conditions
(e.g., hypertension, elevated serum cholesterol level, smoking, and
left ventricular hypertrophy).[40] Part of the reason why the study was
located in Framingham was the fact that the commonwealth of
Massachusetts was supportive and had historically demonstrated a
strong interest in the study of chronic diseases.[41]

According to Thomas R. Dawber, an early director of the study,
and his coauthors, when the study began, "almost nothing was
known" about the "epidemiology of hypertensive or arteriosclerotic
cardiovascular disease."[42] By 1957, based on the findings of the researchers in the Framingham Heart Study, Thomas Dawber and
colleagues published an article in the *American Journal of Public
Health* that described a new risk concept called "multifactorial
causation."[43] Their article showed how several factors could interact to possibly cause heart disease. Hypertension, obesity, and hypercholesteremia were each associated separately with increased
risk of heart disease, but in conjunction with each other, the risk
was even higher. For example, for middle-aged men, the four-year
risk of heart disease was 1% with normal blood pressure and cholesterol, 8% for men with hypertension only, 6% for men with hypercholesteremia only, but 29% for men with both hypertension and

hypercholesteremia, more than the sum of 8% and 6%, even without discounting the reference risk of 1%.[44]

Another approach to the possible causes of cardiovascular diseases compared communities across the world. In 1958, Ancel Keys, a physiologist at the Laboratory of Physiological Hygiene at the University of Minnesota, initiated a formal study of diet, cardiovascular disease risk factors, and heart attack incidence among all men of a given age in sixteen cohorts around the world. These men had a wide range of eating patterns. The Seven Countries Study[45] recruited more than 90 percent of all men who lived in defined rural areas of Finland, Greece, Italy, Japan, Netherlands, the United States, and Yugoslavia.[46] Men in these truly representative samples had comparable rural work activities and social cultures but different dietary habits. Henry Blackburn, a member of the original team, has documented the design and results of the Seven Countries Study on his website Heart Attack Prevention: A History of Cardiovascular Epidemiology.[47]

The study found that the high-fat (mostly from olive oil) and plant-based diet of Greek islanders and the very low-fat diet based on fish and plants in Japan were associated with the lowest rates of heart attacks. In contrast, the incidence of heart attacks was highest in the United States and Finland, where animal fat was highest in the diet. These findings were consistent with the way dietary fatty acids affected serum cholesterol levels in controlled feeding experiments and with the finding of higher cholesterol levels in heart attack victims.[48] The Seven Countries Study contributed to greater understanding of the relationships between diet, blood lipid levels, and heart disease among populations. The epidemiological evidence the study provided and the congruence of that evidence with laboratory and clinical studies has profoundly influenced both preventive practice and overall dietary goals for public health in the United States.

The Seven Countries Study nicely complemented the Framingham Heart Study. It showed that the epidemiological evidence from one small town in Massachusetts was congruent with the evidence from seven rural areas spread across the globe. The determinants of heart attacks that emerged in the Framingham study acted at the population level in the Seven Countries Study. That meant that some of those determinants could possibly also be prevented at the population level.

The Population Strategy of Prevention

Poor diet, obesity, high blood pressure, and high blood cholesterol and glucose levels pose a specific challenge in terms of prevention. In contrast to tobacco consumption, the caloric and nutritional content of the diet, weight, blood cholesterol, and blood pressure cannot be eliminated. They should moderately fluctuate around a safe level. To address this issue, clinicians sought to treat a subgroup of people who were at a high risk of developing cardiovascular diseases. Doctors were eager to know the threshold values that separated safe from unsafe behavioral and biological profiles.

When health care professionals think at the individual level, the damage deleterious behaviors cause seem to primarily affect persons who engage in risk behaviors to excess. Doctors tend to talk to people who drink to excess, people with excessive weight for their height, people with high blood lipids, and so on about what they can do to prevent heart disease. This individual-based medical approach cannot, however, control the burden of heart disease in the population by acting on the subgroup at high risk of developing heart disease.

The switch from an individual to a population approach to preventing diseases caused by specific behaviors began in the 1950s, when demographer Sully Ledermann made some perplexing observations. There were more heavy drinkers in a community if that community drank more alcohol on average than there were in a community that drank less alcohol on average.[49] This was not because of a small group of alcoholic persons pulling the average up. Communities did not seem to be split in two groups of "normal" and heavy drinkers. It was as if excess was more common in communities where the average intake was high. And the opposite was also true: there was less excess in communities where people drank less on average. This observation contradicted the common belief that each society had an immutable core of pathological alcohol drinkers.

Epidemiologist Geoffrey Rose later confirmed Sully Ledermann's observations in an international study that found that the proportion of people who drank more than three glasses of wine per day increased proportionally with the mean level of alcohol consumption.[50] For every additional glass of wine consumed on average, there was an additional 1% of heavy drinkers. More important, if the average intake could be reduced by 10%, there would be 25% fewer heavy drinkers.[51] Rose confirmed Sully Ledermann's observations for issues such as blood pressure, weight-to-height ratio (or body mass index), and salt consumption. In each of these examples, the average exposure predicted the number of persons with excessive risk factors.[52]

Another key observation Rose made was that while high-risk groups may have been much more likely to die from cardiovascular diseases, they represented only a small fraction of the total population.[53] Rose gave the example of the risk of coronary heart disease associated with having a high blood cholesterol in men aged 55–64 years.[54] It is the highest at concentrations at or above 310 mg/100 ml (8 mmol/l), which would be called high ("outside the normal range") by conventional clinical standards. However, only 4% of the population fell in this high-risk category. As a result, less than 10% of the cases of coronary heart disease occurred in this high-risk category. The other 90% arose from the many people who had blood cholesterol within the normal range and who were exposed to a small risk. The implication for public health is that an effective prevention strategy needs to reach the large number of people exposed to a low risk because they produce more cases than a small number of people exposed to a high risk.

Because average behavior impacts the frequency of high-risk behaviors and because most clinical diseases or deaths occur among people whose risk was average, the Public Health Approach would be effective only if its interventions targeted everyone in the population. Rose named this idea the population strategy of prevention, a contrast to the high-risk strategy that would be more typical of the medical approach.[55]

The population strategy of prevention provided additional evidence that a population is a complex superindividual. This way of thinking contrasted with the focus of doctors on individuals who are at high risk for a specific disease. The clinician perspective on the prevention of cardiovascular diseases or cancer is that there are two classes of patients: those (usually a minority) whose behavior is pathological and needs to be modified and those (the majority) whose behavior is normal and does not require any intervention. Why would a physician ask a person who has no extreme behavior or biological traits (e.g., high blood pressure, high blood cholesterol, smoking) to adopt a new diet? In contrast, the population strategy of prevention requires interventions that target everyone. In the second half of the twentieth century, changes in food production and distribution and healthy eating campaigns changed the quality of food products (e.g., meat with lower fat contents) and the buying and eating patterns of consumers. As a likely result, there was a downward trend in cardiovascular diseases in many industrial societies with a Western type of diet.[56]

Both the population-based methodology used to assess the relationship between tobacco consumption and lung cancer and the concept of a population strategy of prevention in the case of cardiovascular diseases have influenced epidemiologists and public health officials enormously. With the population-based method for causal inference and the population strategy of prevention, the

Public Health Approach was well equipped to search for the cause of cancers and cardiovascular diseases and to intervene at the population level to reduce their prevalence. However, it was not ready for the emergence of new infectious diseases with pandemic characteristics. The Public Health Approach did not yet have the statistical tools it needed to cope with HIV/AIDS.

Chapter 7

HIV/AIDS

In June 1981, the *Morbidity and Mortality Weekly Report*, the journal of the Centers for Disease Control and Prevention, reported that five cases of *pneumocystis carinii pneumonia* had been identified among young gay men in California. Almost simultaneously, an unusually malignant form of skin cancer, Kaposi's sarcoma, was diagnosed in the United States, also among gay men.[1] Both diseases were opportunistic infections, illnesses that are typical among immunocompromised persons but that a healthy immune system can neutralize. It was later understood that these were the first manifestations of a new pandemic. The Human Immunodeficiency Virus (HIV) had been originally transmitted to humans from nonhuman primates in the 1930s. The earliest known case of HIV-1 was a patient in Kinshasa, Zaire, in 1959. The virus became pandemical in the 1980s, when most patients were infected by the HIV-1 strain or the less common HIV-2 strain. The first manifestations were opportunistic infections because the 10 billion new HIV viral particles per day have the ability to overwhelm the cells that protect from infections by *pneumocystis carinii* or by the Kaposi sarcoma–associated herpesvirus.[2]

In 1982 already, it was established that 75% of the cases of these immunodeficiency-related diseases in the first years of the pandemic occurred in homosexual or bisexual males.[3] Most of the remaining 25% had no history of male homosexual activity. Many were intravenous drug users, Haitians residing in the United States, or had received blood transfusions for hemophilia. Uncertainty reigned for more than two years about the origin of AIDS. Was it caused by an infectious or by a behavioral disease? The saga of how medical researchers determined that the disease was caused by a virus is narrated in the book and movie *And the Band Played On*.

While virologists were slow in identifying the virus, because it killed the cells in which they tried to cultivate it, epidemiologists could have had an opportunity to detect an association that explained why unrelated communities were affected. But that didn't happen. A strictly viral origin of the syndrome seemed implausible in 1981 and 1982. Almost forty years of epidemiological research that had focused on cancer and cardiovascular disease had generated a method for identifying modifiable factors such as tobacco consumption, diet, drug use, and occupational exposures.[4] Epidemiologists began searching for exposures that could depress the immune response, alone or in conjunction with a microorganism such as a cytomegalovirus. We now know that attempts to link recreational drugs (e.g., amyl nitrite, a substance that improved the experience of anal intercourse) or therapeutic drugs (e.g., anal use of corticoid creams) were ill founded, particularly because it was known very early on that the syndrome affected other populations besides gay men.[5] This pursuit ended in May 1983, when a team of virologists reported that they had identified the AIDS virus, a T-lymphotropic retrovirus.[6]

Even though diagnostic tests quickly became available, in the 1980s HIV infections were too rare in Western societies to permit mass screening. Because of the small rate of error associated with the test and the low prevalence of the infection, there would have been too many false positive tests. The belief then was that mass screening would have caused unbearable stress for people falsely suspected to have HIV/AIDS until they received the results of a blood test that was developed in 1985, which confirmed or disconfirmed the screening test. In a mass screening scenario, the results of the first screening test would be confirmed by a Western blot test that assessed the body's immune response to specific HIV proteins.[7] Instead of pursuing mass testing, the focus was on informing the public about the preventive behaviors that worked: practicing safe sex.

Once the virus was isolated, the search for a vaccine and a treatment began. The HIV/AIDS epidemic enriched the Public Health Approach by contributing to the development of a way to assess the efficacy of antiviral treatment that solved methodological challenges that had been unsolvable until then.

Treatment by Indication

In medical practice, when a drug becomes available for a specific disease, it is likely to be prescribed preferentially to patients who are in life-threatening conditions and who are therefore likely to succumb from the disease. As a result, a larger proportion of those who get the drug die compared to those who don't get it. A comparison of two groups of patients, one receiving the drug and the other not, may give the impression that the drug is not effective, but that is only because those who were treated had a worse prognosis to begin with. This spurious result is caused by a type of study bias called treatment by indication because the treatment is given to the patients suffering from the most severe forms of the disease.

The epidemiological methods that had been developed to study cancer and cardiovascular diseases were not ready to disentangle associations potentially affected by the treatment by indication bias. Typically, when studying cancer and cardiovascular diseases the exposure to the postulated cause, such as high blood pressure or cigarette smoking, was measured at a fixed moment in time that was considered to be a baseline. The outcome of interest, such as coronary heart disease or lung cancer, was assessed one time during the period after the baseline when the groups that had been exposed were at risk of developing that outcome. That is known as the risk period. The association required a single causal arrow: $T \to Y$, where T is an exposure and Y is an outcome. Conventional methods of adjusting for differences between the compared groups under this simple associational scheme do not eliminate bias created by treatment by indication.[8]

In the mid-1970s, researchers in the human and social sciences were exploring ways of designing nonrandomized studies to make their participants as comparable as if they had been randomized.[9] Was there a way to create groups in a nonrandomized study that would be as similar as they would have been if the exposure had been allocated using a chance-based procedure? In their quest, these researchers built a theory based on our intuitive perception of what a cause is at an individual level. Consider these statements: "Had I been vaccinated against SARS-CoV-2 a month ago instead of hesitating, I would not have gotten COVID-19 now." Or "because I was vaccinated against SARS-CoV-2 a month ago and did not hesitate, I did not get COVID-19 now." Intuitively, we compare what has happened with what would have happened had we acted differently.[10] The comparison is strictly hypothetical. A person was vaccinated against SARS-CoV-2 and did not get COVID-19 for the next six months. It is not possible to go back in time and, in the first statement, inject the vaccine, or, in the second statement, inject an inactive fluid (a placebo) instead of the vaccine in the arm of this same person and observe what happens, as if life could be lived twice, once after receiving the vaccine and once after receiving the placebo. The only comparative option at the individual level, studying the effect of the vaccine with everything else being identical, requires that a life is lived twice, under two different exposure scenarios, which is impossible. The causal question, about whether the vaccine works, therefore has no solution at the individual level. But a solution is possible when the perspective shifts to the population level and when some conditions related to the research topic and the experiment are met.

In public health, these ideas were first applied to an apparently intractable problem in occupational health, analogous to treatment by indication bias, before being used successfully to evaluate the efficacy of treatment against HIV/AIDS. I will therefore first explain the problem of the healthy worker bias and its solution before returning to the application of that solution to the assessment of whether an early anti-HIV drug was effective in slowing the progression toward AIDS.

Healthy Worker Bias

In the mid-1980s, epidemiologist James Robins theorized that the causal thinking proposed by Donald Rubin described above was appropriate for handling situations analogous to the treatment by indication bias. Say that workers who have been exposed to a particular toxic chemical at work are at an increased risk of cancer. Those who terminate their employment because they have become ill have been exposed to the toxic chemical for a shorter time than workers who do not get sick and continue to work.[11]

Robins reanalyzed the all-cause and lung cancer mortality experience of a cohort of arsenic-exposed copper smelter workers. Copper extraction from mined arsenic-containing ores involves a process of heating that releases gaseous arsenic which smelters inhales and can cause cancers. There were 5,947 arsenic-exposed white males who were hired subsequent to January 1, 1935, at a Montana copper smelter and worked there for at least one year until 1956. From date of hire to end of follow-up in 1977 there were 1,784 deaths, of which 116 were due to lung cancer. Jobs had different levels of arsenic exposure.[12]

Robins first used the conventional method, based on the simple, single-arrowed model, $T \rightarrow Y$, where T is exposure to arsenic and Y is all-cause mortality. The workers more exposed were not at greater risk of dying than those with a lower arsenic exposure. There did not seem to be an adverse effect of arsenic on total mortality. Robins then compared these results with those of the new method compatible with the work of Rubin described above and found an adverse effect of arsenic exposure that standard methods fail to detect.

The reason for this discrepancy between the conventional and the new model was that those remaining on the job are a priori healthier than those who had to leave work and therefore abbreviate their total exposure to arsenic. Robins pointed out that when studying the health effects of arsenic, a simple comparison of the workers remaining on the job might incorrectly infer that the workers who are exposed for a longer period are safe; they are apparently as likely to become sick as those who were exposed for a shorter period but got sick and interrupted their exposure to arsenic. In reality, the workers who stayed on the job remained free of disease because for some reason they were healthier and more resistant to the exposure. This is called the healthy worker bias, what Robins referred to as "occupational exposures [that are] masked by the early termination of workers with poor prognosis."[13] In this type of bias, the true level of risk of the workers can be misestimated.

Even in an ultra-simplified model (fig. 7.1), the core of the association between arsenic and death requires multiple arrows: T is the exposure to arsenic at two points in time, M is the employment status (yes or no) at two points in time, and Y is death.

To analyze situations such as that represented in figure 7.1, Robins offered a solution based on the idea of observing the same individual twice: once when they are exposed to the chemical and again if they had not been exposed. The impossible design at the individual level can be simulated at the population level, as if every worker

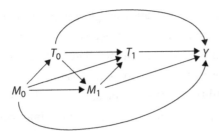

FIGURE 7.1. Diagram of the relation between a treatment T and an outcome Y, given markers M of the severity of the treated disease. Two points in time are indicated by the subscripts 0 and 1.

in the study would have had two lives.[14] One life in which they would all have continually high exposure to arsenic and one life in which their exposure to arsenic would have been continually low, everything else staying the same. The time of these sustained exposures mattered. The whole study sample functions now as a superindividual. How many deaths would have been observed if this superindividual, whether the workers it comprised stayed on or left work, had had a high exposure? Inversely, how many deaths would have been observed if the superindividual, whether they stayed on or left work, had had a low exposure? Because the same population is compared to itself, under two hypothetical scenarios, the healthy worker bias does not operate.

Figure 7.1 does not get at the real brilliance of Robins's model, which enriched the Public Health Approach by showing how to analyze the effect of a cause the exposure to which changes over time. This was an important issue that previous methods developed to study the causes of lung cancer and cardiovascular disease had not considered. Robins showed how to bring together information on exposure and other factors that vary across time. In addition, the superindividual is not just exposed versus unexposed at different moments of its existence. It has other characteristics that change over time such as age, job titles, employment, smoking history, and so on. All these time-varying characteristics continuously influence each other, and they need to be included in the analysis in order to isolate the effect of the exposure to arsenic. In the end, if some important conditions are met, the study based on observing what happened to a population of workers across time will measure the same effect of arsenic on health as if the workers had been randomized to be continually exposed to high vs low concentrations of gaseous arsenic. Since randomizing exposure to arsenic is unreasonable, the methods developed by Robins offered the only option to assess the occupational health effects of arsenic.

AZT Treatment for AIDS

Soon after AIDS emerged as a potential epidemic disease, a modified version of zidovudine (AZT), a failed anti-cancer drug, was found to inhibit the action of the virus. The US Food and Drug Administration (FDA), under great pressure from the public, fast-tracked its review of the drug in March 1987.[15]

Randomized trials immediately began to assess the efficacy of AZT for slowing down the progression of AIDS or preventing death.[16] However, researchers conducting the trials faced challenges. For example, because AZT, but not the placebo, caused severe intestinal problems, nausea, vomiting and headaches, participants could guess that they were assigned to the control group and would drop out if they could get access to AZT in some other way. There was, however, a great deal of information available about people who were getting AZT whether or not they were participating in trials. The need to correctly analyze these randomized and nonrandomized data became urgent.

There were several methodological challenges to designing a nonrandomized trial for AZT. The HIV-positive persons who were receiving the drug were not comparable to participants who were not receiving it because of the treatment by indication bias discussed above: the treatment tended to be prescribed for sicker patients. Since those people were sicker when they began the treatment, a disproportionate number of participants in the treatment groups died. Moreover, doctors changed the dosages they prescribed for a patient each time the disease flared up, according to the fluctuating levels of white blood cell count or in response to the side effects the drug and/or the severity of the disease. Epidemiological methods that could accommodate these study conditions were not being taught in the leading schools of public health at that time.

James Robins noted that the underlying difficulty of AZT trials was the same as the difficulty that produced the healthy worker bias: in the AZT trials, people were being treated by indication, and factors that determined treatment were changing over time. He applied his model for addressing this particular type of bias in an article titled "Analysis of Randomized and Nonrandomized AIDS Treatment Trials Using a New Approach to Causal Inference in Longitudinal Studies."[17] The diagram in figure 7.1 also applies to the association of AZT and AIDS. In this case the dosage of treatment T depends on the markers M of the severity of the disease in the patient, (e.g., white blood cell count, drug side effects, clinical signs). Both T and M at time 0 and time 1 impact the outcome Y, which in the case of AIDS can be relapse or death.

The methodology Robins developed for analyzing AIDS treatment data helped to solve many other questions about causation that could not be answered with the methods inherited from studies of the association between, for example, tobacco and lung cancer.[18] Robins's method is now used in much health and social science research, including epidemiology, and is taught in textbooks.[19]

Thus, the deadly HIV/AIDS pandemic appears to have accelerated the integration of a new conceptual framework that resulted in the refinement of the Public Health Approach. The perspective switch consisted of adapting an individual-based definition of causality to the study of a population using a study design that viewed the entire study sample as a superindividual, and the data from that superindividual could be statistically manipulated to approximate the outcome as if all study participants had been both exposed to a treatment and not.

Chapter 8

Social Determinants of Health

Until the last decades of the twentieth century, the Public Health Approach was mainly used in the context of controlling epidemics of infectious diseases and for urging people to modify unhealthy behaviors suspected to cause noninfectious diseases. Consuming tobacco and eating a diet rich in animal products and poor in fruits and vegetables were targeted as causes of the epidemics of cancer and cardiovascular diseases. These diseases had been of marginal importance in human societies before the twentieth century. It looked like these diseases were consequences of the modern way of life.

However, the modern way of life did not impact every stratum of society in the same way. It soon became apparent that not everyone has the means to make the changes that constitute a healthy lifestyle. As a result, public health researchers began to pay more attention to the health consequences of unequal access to essential human needs such as housing, food, health, clothing, education, and justice. In other words, public health researchers began to tackle the social determinants of health,[1] which involved "making the invisible causes of population health visible."[2] Social determinants of health are aspects of the economy, education, health care, and people's social and built environments that affect their health, functioning, and quality of life.[3]

Some people think about the social determinants of health in individualistic terms. They believe that poverty is the fault of the poor or that school achievement is solely attributable to a student's dedication to schoolwork and their innate intelligence. Social norms, laws, institutions, and policies are often based on beliefs about who is "good" and who is "bad" within a society. Such thinking can be extended to entire ethnic groups, for example by associating alleged psychological or physical traits with skin color. These speculative explanations do not cohere with what is scientifically known about how populations react to social and economic stressors.

Historian Alan Derickson reported an example of the latter type of thinking in "'A Widespread Superstition': The Purported Invulnerability of Workers of Color to Occupational Heat Stress."[4] He described how American slave owners believed that workers of African descent could tolerate extreme temperatures because of their physical constitution and how advocates of racial segregation in tropical colonies argued that Chinese immigrants should do the strenuous work that whites were not constitutionally able to do. Farmers in the US South also claimed that Mexican immigrants who did agricultural work were naturally suited for unhealthful working conditions.

The construction of the Hoover Dam across the Colorado River in 1931–1936 was an accidental population experiment that debunked speculative arguments that the genetic background of some populations meant that they had been naturally selected to fit them for inhuman environmental conditions. Workers on the Hoover Dam project were required to work outdoors in the Sonoran

Desert in extreme heat. Because of the Great Depression, the managers of the project hired unemployed white workers and discriminated against workers of color; only a few Black workers were hired. The team of mostly white workers built an engineering marvel under temperatures that reached 130° Fahrenheit or 54° Celsius, enough heat to cook a steak rare. This project conclusively proved that white workers are also capable of laboring in extreme environmental conditions.[5]

The civil rights movement of the 1960s challenged the theories that argued that there existed ethnic, constitutional differences in population health. Movement activists, researchers, and academics showed that there was a pattern in access to housing, food, health care, clothing, education, and justice that disadvantaged entire communities. Activists in the social and political movements of the 1960s promoted the idea that health is a human right.[6] The struggle for the rights of workers, members of disadvantaged communities, members of sexual minorities, citizens of colonized nations, and many more groups was linked to health inequities that served as a practical indicator of the fairness of a society. Sociologist Alondra Nelson has described the key role of community health work in Black activism from slavery times to the Black Lives Matter movement.[7]

Since the 1960s, many people have challenged the ideology of individual or ethnic responsibility and criticized how societies produce injustice and inequalities. They switched perspectives. The belief in individual responsibility is a form of victim blaming. An example is the argument that people with few economic options are to blame for being mistreated by the police or that unemployed workers are to blame for becoming drug addicts. Many people now reject the concept of individual responsibility because they recognize that the causes of many disadvantages are social. This chapter discusses two examples of health issues that are socially determined instead of being caused by individual heredity or individual susceptibility: the disproportionate incidence of police brutality against and incarceration of people of color and the decline in the life expectancy of middle-aged US whites.

Police and Prisons

From an individual perspective, police violence may appear to be the implementation of the law to punish minor and major offenses. Each brutalized person and each incarcerated person can be associated with specific contexts. However, when statistics about police violence are analyzed by skin color, it immediately becomes apparent that people of color suffer violent attacks by police in numbers that are disproportionate to their percentage of the US population.

Mapping Police Violence is a project that uses data from local and state government agencies, from university initiatives such as Fatal Encounters,[8] and from publicly available media sources. The group believes that its website provides "the most comprehensive accounting of people killed by police since 2013."[9] From 2013 to 2021, US police killed 4,347 white people (50.5% of the total of 8,613 people killed among white, Black, and Hispanic victims), 2,491 Black people (28.9%), and 1,775 Hispanic people (20.6%). Every year police killed approximately 500 whites, 300 blacks and 200 Hispanics (fig. 8.1).

When we look at these numbers, it seems like white people are at the highest risk of being killed in an encounter with police. How can we reconcile that perception with the widespread press coverage of police killings of people of color such as Trayvon Martin, Eric Garner, Freddie Gray, Breonna Taylor, Andres Guardado, Michael Brown, Tamir Rice, Walter Scott, Carlos Lopez, Alton Sterling Philando Castile, Jamar Clark, George Floyd, and Sandra Bland? The coverage seems disproportionate to the fact that fewer people of color are killed than white people every year.

But when we look at police killings in the United States from a population standpoint, the perspective changes. When the number of killings by racial or ethnic group is compared to the number of

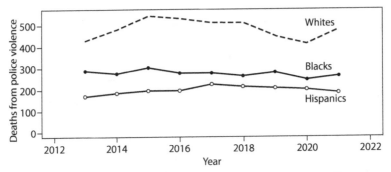

FIGURE 8.1. Number of Black, Hispanic, and white people killed by US police, 2013–2021. There is a striking regularity in the trends showing that the police killed approximately 500 whites, 300 Blacks, and 200 Hispanic every year between 2013 and 2021. https://mappingpoliceviolence.org/.

people in that group in the general population of the United States, a pattern becomes clear.[10] In the period 2013–2021, police killed Black people at a much higher rate than white people (fig. 8.2). The average yearly rate of Black people killed at the hands of police per million Black people in the United States over those nine years was 6.8.[11] In contrast, the number of white people killed in police encounters per million white people in the United States is 2.5. Police killed Black people during that decade at a rate that was 2.7 times higher than the rate at which they killed white people. Other racial/ethnic groups are targeted at higher rates than whites: Native Americans were killed at a rate that was 1.7 times higher than that of whites, and Hispanic people were killed at a rate 1.3 times higher than that of whites. The population perspective of looking at the rate of deaths per million people in each racial/ethnic group reveals a disparity in how police interact with Black people and other people of color. This is an example of a social determinant of health, in this case of survival.[12]

The pattern has been extremely stable since 2013 (fig. 8.2). Relative to the size of each community, Blacks are killed more frequently by police officers than whites.[13] The pattern suggests supraindividual

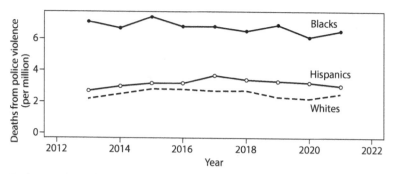

FIGURE 8.2. Rates (per million per year) of Black, Hispanic, and white persons killed by US police, 2013–2021. https://mappingpoliceviolence.org/.

causes that can be studied and identified using a Public Health Approach. For years, articles in the *American Journal of Public Health* have been stressing the importance of systematically documenting these killings and their impact on public health. This mass phenomenon can impact the health of entire communities at the physical, mental, and economic level.

Mass incarceration also requires a population perspective in order to see the racial pattern. As of August 18, 2022, 157,739 people were incarcerated in federal prisons.[14] Of this population, 38.4% (60,441) were Black and 57.6% (90,788) were white. The percentage of incarcerated Black people is disproportionate to their representation within the US population: Black Americans represent 13% of the general US population but 38% of people in prison or jail. Another way to see the racial pattern is to look at the rate of incarceration per 100,000 people within a racial or ethnic group. The overall incarceration rate for Black people is 2,306 per 100,000 members of that group in the total US population. The corresponding figure for white Americans is 450 per 100,000. Blacks are incarcerated 5.12 times more often than whites.[15]

"Black people are more likely to be arrested, killed by police, incarcerated, and placed in solitary confinement than their White counterparts," Lauren Brinkley-Rubinstein and David Cloud wrote to 64 years in counties with only small or medium-sized cities and in rural areas. They were dying more from self-inflicted harm such as suicide, drug overdoses, poisoning, and alcohol-related liver disease. Case and Deaton referred to this epidemic of self-destructive behaviors as evidence of the "deaths of despair."[20] The expression has now become common usage, even though there is no definitive proof that it accurately describes the underlying phenomenon.

These deaths have been explained by the loss of low-tech manufacturing jobs since the 1980s and the stagnation of wage rates.[21] One narrative points to the fact that white workers with a limited education who were unable to get good-paying jobs with good benefits are failing economically and socially compared to their parents. Joblessness decimated trade union membership and weakened union strength and networks. Increased poverty may have weakened family, community, or religious support. The overall consequence has been despair and depression following the weakening of institutions that can deter individuals from harming themselves.[22]

Declines in life expectancy are rare. In the past, they have occurred after major pandemics or in times of unusual levels of economic hardship. For example, life expectancy decreased in the Soviet Union after its collapse in 1991 as a result of a 40 percent surge in deaths from all causes between 1990 and 1994.[23] These are extreme circumstances. Case and Deaton discovered a phenomenon that was unanticipated because it affected a white majority during a period when the entire country wasn't experiencing extreme hardship. The phenomenon was striking at the population level but was imperceptible at the individual level. One reason why the phenomenon escaped even standard health monitoring techniques may be that the relative magnitude of the deaths of despair were small compared to the overall differences in life expectancy for all Blacks and all whites. Stein and her colleagues found that, overall, in 2013–2015, Blacks had an excess mortality compared to whites of +152 per 100,000, which is about ten times larger than the +15 per 100,000 excess deaths over fifteen years for suburban and rural whites aged 25 to 64.[24]

Structural Racism

A striking commonality of inequities in incarceration rates and the deaths of despair is that they haven't had major public health policy consequences. This may be due in part to the fact that the Public Health Approach to social determinants of health still needs to build up its scientific basis and translate its findings into policy.

Violence against People of Color

A Public Health Approach to police brutality needs to go beyond videos that attest to its existence but not to its extent. Scientific, consistent, comprehensive documentation is the first step toward establishing the scientific evidence that can guide policy. Video releases and press coverage of specific crimes may reveal only the tip of the iceberg. The lack of comprehensive data may hide the nature and the magnitude of the problem at the population level.

A first question is how to assess police brutality, which includes all conduct that dehumanizes and degrades victims. Sirry Alang and colleagues have proposed five consequences of police brutality that lead to excess illness among Blacks at both the individual and the community level: fatal injuries; increased morbidity; stress; arrests, incarcerations, and legal, medical, and funeral bills that cause financial strain; and systematic disempowerment.[25]

There is increasing awareness that the time is ripe for major reforms that could prevent police brutality and significantly reduce incarcerations. Some obvious reforms can be enacted and evaluated immediately. For example, reallocating resources to nonrepressive forms of community service may enable unarmed social and community health workers, like the interrupters of Safe Streets in Baltimore,[26] to address issues that arise because of depression, inadequate housing, addiction, and compromised mental health. However, to date, good intentions have rarely been translated into action.

History shows that there is no effective shortcut that can produce the results and analysis that comes out of careful studies that record all events and examine the sources and impact of violence on all social groups. Such studies can provide the basis for science-based policies. Police brutality and mass incarceration are social problems with structural causes that lead to health inequities. Funding for science and community service that is backed by political support will help researchers understand these structural causes and ideally lead to policies that will dismantle the social determinants of health that are causing so much harm.

Deaths of Despair

One can speculate that whites have a greater risk than Blacks of being depressed by the lack of a good job because of centuries of racial privilege. Even though the theory sounds reasonable, until it is supported by experimental evidence, it won't be of much use for public health. The hypothesis merits comparative studies that may provide evidence that the apparent link is a causal one. Other social groups have been impacted by the shrinking of the workforce in the auto, steel, coal, textile and other industries that thrived in the 1950s and 1960s and were sources of good jobs for both men and women.[27]

Is it possible to understand the recent negative trend in the life expectancy of some groups of white people independently from the chronic but steady excess mortality of Black Americans? The decline in white life expectancy is dwarfed by the magnitude of the racial inequities that cause excess mortality for Black people. In addition, the deindustrialization that impacted whites also impacted Black workers. The decline of the industrial core of the American economy has literally eliminated the Black industrial working class in the Appalachian region and beyond.[28] Why haven't Black workers experienced the decrease in life expectancy that white workers have? What is the role of mass incarceration and police violence in the mortality rate by "deaths of despair" of Black Americans? What is the link between mass incarceration and mass unemployment among Black workers? The gendered dimension of the deaths of despair theory, which focuses on white men, is perplexing: some observations indicate that the increase in death rates among whites may be more pronounced in women than in men.[29] Chetty and co-authors argue that geography is highly correlated with the differences in the mortality rates of the rich and the poor.[30] There is also evidence that despair indicators have been rising among US adults who have been entering midlife since 2010 and that increases in early mortality are not concentrated among white, low-educated, rural adults.[31] Finally, analysis of midlife mortality rates in the United States up to 2016 shows that increases have been driven by a wide range of conditions in addition to factors related to despair. Professor of population health Steven H. Woolf and his colleagues note that these conditions affect all racial and ethnic groups: "The wide range of affected conditions points to the need to examine systemic causes of declining health in the US."[32]

A Single Public Health Problem?

In part, the chronic excess mortality among people of color compared to whites may be the result of the same economic and social conditions that are allegedly responsible for the "deaths of despair." They call for strategies that can foster a sense of belonging, meaning, and hope and promote healthy behaviors.

As Shanahan and colleagues explain, conceptually mapping the associations between social determinants of health and their suspected health outcome, identifying whether "despair" is indeed a common pathway to several causes of death, and testing them may

Chapter 9

The 1918 Influenza and SARS/COVID-19

Ever since the H1N1 virus that caused 20–60 million deaths in a world population of 1.8 billion in 1918, public health officials had been expecting another global pandemic. The SARS-CoV-2 virus caused that event. In 1918, most people on the planet lived in rural areas. When the H1N1 estimates are adjusted for the increase in the world's population, a scourge of similar magnitude would have killed 80 to 240 million people in 2020. In comparison, the World Health Organization has estimated that COVID-19 killed 3 million people in 2020 of a world population that was an estimated 7.6 billion at the beginning of that year.[1] Densely populated metropolitan areas facilitated the spread of infection. In 1918, the H1N1 virus was new for humans and unfolded in an immunologically naïve population. The same was true as the COVID-19 epidemic unfolded in 2020.

Lessons of 1918

In 1918, scientists could not tell for sure whether the culprit was a virus or which virus it was. Ideas about disease transmission and person-to-person contamination of the flu were primitive. It was the end of World War I, and the virus was traveling back and forth across the oceans in packed army ships.[2] It spread across regiments in barracks that were incompatible with physical distancing, hand washing, and other forms of hygiene in a context in which nonpharmaceutical interventions such as closing schools, restricting public gatherings, and isolation and quarantine were the only available responses.

Despite these very difficult conditions, the United States Public Health Service conducted a large survey from November 20, 1918, to March 12, 1919, to assess the incidence rate and mortality of the influenza pandemic among 146,203 persons in eighteen localities across the United States.[3] It was a huge endeavor. The survey included a house-to-house canvass in the eighteen regions to arrive at a fair sample of the general population. As soon as possible after the epidemic appeared to have definitely subsided, survey employees interviewed a responsible member of every household in the selected areas.

The Public Health Service survey provides unique population-based information about the magnitude of the pandemic in the United States. The prevalence of symptomatic influenza over six months was 29.4%, ranging from 15% in Louisville, Kentucky, to 53.3% in San Antonio, Texas. The overall percentage of deaths among the infected was 1.70%, ranging from 0.78% in San Antonio to 3.14% in New London, Connecticut. These results were based on self-reports of symptoms. Assuming that the survey missed one-third of cases due to infected people who were asymptomatic,[4] it is likely that over 50% of Americans were infected and about 1% of those who were infected died.[5]

Since that catastrophe, scientists repeatedly warned that a new pandemic was pending. The only question was when. Alarms about potentially catastrophic outbreaks happened numerous times. Examples include the swine flu in 1976, against which President Gerald

Ford ordered a mass vaccination,[6] and the bird flu scare of 2005, an outbreak of H5N1 avian influenza, against which the government stockpiled Tamiflu, a modestly effective antiviral drug.[7] Both in 1976 and in 2005, the vaccination mandates were fiascos that can serve as referents to gauge the accomplishments of the COVID-19 vaccination campaign.

In November 2018, an issue of the *American Journal of Public Health* that commemorated 100 years since the 1918 flu described the social context of that event, which in hindsight predicted the events that unfolded during the SARS-CoV-2/COVID-19 pandemic. Opinions diverged about whether the world was prepared to control a similar scourge and avoid a humanitarian disaster. Counterterrorism and emergency response expert Michael Greenberger argued that the United States was not prepared and was following a cycle of "panic-neglect-panic-neglect" in its approach to pandemics.[8] Nurse researcher Barbara Jester and her colleagues from the CDC believed that the United States was prepared even though there were areas where we could improve.[9] They stressed that public health laboratories could detect seasonal, novel, and emerging pandemic influenza viruses in the United States much earlier and more accurately than in the past and that a vaccine could be rapidly produced. Dr. Jason Schwartz argued that nonpharmaceutical interventions, such as closing schools and public gathering places or separating infected or exposed people from their communities would remain prominent features of epidemic response strategies.[10] Mark A. Rothstein and Wendy Parmet concluded that the United States was better off in 2018 than it had been in 1918, but that we were still vulnerable because of major gaps in our preparedness plans:

A third problem is distrust. In our era of political polarization, "fake news," and tribal politics, trust in the media, government officials, and even science is fading. This can be catastrophic if an influenza or another type of pandemic arises. Under such circumstances, the public's failure to trust the guidance offered by public health officials may well make a bad situation worse.[11]

The information in some of the articles in the commemorative issue was scary. The authors were experts who had long experience with issues of counterterrorism, cybersecurity, and catastrophic health events such as seasonal flu, the Ebola virus, the Zika virus, and the opioids epidemic. The consensus was that despite enormous technological and scientific breakthroughs since 1918, preparedness plans were inadequate. The authors hoped that a catastrophic scenario could be prevented if a universal vaccine could be rapidly produced after the characteristics of a new virus were identified. They stressed that during the next epidemic or pandemic, there would be an urgent need for a bipartisan information campaign about the safety of the vaccine in order to preempt fake news and provide information about the importance of vaccination.

Before the first case of COVID-19 occurred, governments around the world knew that a dreadful pandemic, probably of influenza, was inevitable. Scientists knew how it would unfold and that the vaccine would be an essential component of the response. There was plenty of time to prepare for another pandemic, yet the US government did not do it. In fact, the United States reduced its preparedness resources and marginalized its experts in the period 2001–2019. During those two decades, government spending and appropriations for public health decreased,[12] and the resources, independence, and scientific authority of the CDC were reduced. In 2018, the National Security Council Directorate for Global Health Security and Biodefense was eliminated; it had been created in 2014 to coordinate the response of federal agencies to the Ebola outbreak and other global disasters.[13] At the population level, adjustments in the management of the Affordable Care Act (ACA, also known as Obamacare) after 2016 decreased access to health care and increased the number of uninsured people.[14] In 2019, Kathryn E. W. Himmelstein and Atheendar S. Venkataramani calculated that approximately 1 million health care workers were uninsured and therefore impeded from taking care of their own health in case of a pandemic.[15] During the COVID-19 pandemic, fear that cooperating with public health officials would lead to arrest or deportation hindered some immigrants from cooperating with quarantine directives.[16] Most undocumented immigrants are also excluded from public health programs such as Medicaid and fear that seeking health care will reveal their status to government officials. Legal scholars Mark Rothstein and Christine Coughlin predicted in 2019 that these factors "may worsen public health outcomes in an epidemic unless [the] unique needs [of undocumented immigrants] are considered when formulating public health policy."[17]

Despite these obstacles, the epidemiological and biomedical responses to COVID-19 ended up in my view being extremely consequential. When the pandemic broke out, epidemiologists and other population scientists reacted swiftly.[18] They quickly described the cause and the evolution of the pandemic. As early as January 2020, publications were forecasting the potential domestic and international spread of the outbreak that was discovered in Wuhan, China.[19] In the following weeks, scientists showed that physical distancing, masking, and confinement or quarantine were effective; that older age groups were at the highest risk; that there was a four-day latency period between infection and clinical symptoms; and that asymptomatic cases were contagious. These and many more key scientific findings enabled governments around the world to make decisions to order lockdowns and to recommend social distancing and the use of personal protective equipment.

Scientists quickly evaluated the efficacy of potential treatments. During the first year, most drug candidates for treating COVID-19 were shown to be ineffective. The mass assessment of the Pfizer vaccine in Israel and later of the vaccines of other companies proved that they were highly effective.

The development of vaccines and the mass vaccination campaigns were both remarkable achievements. Urgently reaching hundreds of millions of Americans who wanted to be vaccinated is a challenge that had never been met before. It required coordination between the federal government and state and local health departments. The vaccine coverage in the United States may be lower than in some other wealthy countries, but it was an extraordinary performance in US public health history.

However, no surveillance system was in place to track the dissemination of the pandemic, the speed at which it infected people, and who was primarily infected. This was one of the greatest failures of the Public Health Approach response to COVID-19.

Flying Blind

Since 2020, the progression of the pandemic has not been adequately tracked in the United States. A modern health monitoring system is missing. Such a system, which relies on repeated representative sampling of diverse parts of the population, is still not in place for future pandemics. Its absence complicated the policy responses to SARS-CoV-2, especially in terms of identifying which communities were most affected and making decisions about lockdowns of schools and businesses.

There is no substitute for data that is collected for the specific purposes of tracking the progress of a pandemic and determining whether countermeasures are slowing the pandemic down. In the absence of a system for collecting these data, the government, the public, and the press had to interpret reports from hospitals and health centers of the numbers of people who had decided to get tested or were so sick that they ended up in a hospital, where their case was recorded.[20] These samples were highly selected and did not reflect the true progression of the virus. Data about numbers of cases often lacked information on ethnicity and race. Officials lacked evidence about what proportion of the population was infected, what proportion of the infected was asymptomatic, and which communities were most affected.

In an article titled "Inside America's COVID-Reporting Breakdown," health care reporter Erin Banco used the expression that is the subheading of this section: "Covid-19 was spreading rapidly throughout the United States, as cold winter weather began to drive people indoors, but the Centers for Disease Control and Prevention was flying blind: The state agencies that it relied on were way behind in their tracking, with numbers trickling in from labs by fax or even snail mail."[21]

In an interview with the *Wall Street Journal*, CDC director Rochelle Walensky acknowledged that the data collection system is inadequate:

> Fewer than 200 health facilities across the U. S. had their electronic-health records linked to CDC data-collection systems before the pandemic, Dr. Walensky said. At the start of the pandemic, some states that were unable to electronically report positive COVID-19 cases had to fax PCR results to the CDC, she said. Some states were entering positive results first because they didn't have the capacity to enter all the negative ones, she said, so the CDC initially received a skewed view of what fraction of the population was positive.[22]

The lack of accurate statistics on COVID-19 created a dilemma even for the *American Journal of Public Health*. Should analyses based on inaccurate data be published to document, even imperfectly, the impact of the pandemic? Alternatively, should findings that could overestimate or underestimate its true impact and thus be contradicted later be barred from publication? As a rule, the journal does not publish the results of surveys that do not comply with statistical criteria of representativeness. Should the journal have made an exception for COVID-19? There was huge pressure from authors to do so and report how different communities were affected. The journal decided to stand by its pre-COVID-19 policy. It published a paper by four senior epidemiologists, Neal Pearce, Jan Vandenbroucke, Tyler Vander Wiele, and Sander Greenland, that explained the criteria for the validity of such statistics.[23]

In public media, very basic claims such as reports that the United States was "the epicenter" of the pandemic because it had more cases than places like Italy ignored the fact that the US population is over five times larger than that of Italy. Most important, Neil Pearce and colleagues summarized the characteristics that an ideal surveillance system would need in order to generate locally reliable and internationally comparable data:

1. repeated representative sampling of diverse parts of the population;
2. screening/diagnostic test performance and validation for each brand, laboratory, and country; and
3. estimates of fatality rates among those who tested positive for infection based on representative samples of the population who have been followed for a sufficient length of time.[24]

The reality in the United States was very far from that ideal.

The absence of a population-based national dashboard was partly responsible for the grim side of the pandemic response in the United States. The US suffered the highest death rate of any wealthy country, and the impact was unfair and unjust. The expression

"We're all in this together" irritated psychologist Lisa Bowleg, who wrote:

> Although seemingly innocuous and often well intentioned, the phrase reflects an intersectional color- and class-blinding that functions to obscure the structural inequities that befall Black and other marginalized groups, who bear the harshest and most disproportionate brunt of anything negative or calamitous: HIV/AIDS, hypertension, poverty, diabetes, climate change disasters, unemployment, mass incarceration, and, now, COVID-19.[25]

In the summer of 2020, Nancy Krieger wrote an editorial in the *American Journal of Public Health* titled "ENOUGH: COVID-19, Structural Racism, Police Brutality, Plutocracy, Climate Change—and Time for Health Justice, Just Governance, and an Equitable, Sustainable Future."[26] The title is a mouthful, but its message is clear: structural inequalities enabled the virus to thrive in the US population. In 2020, there was a public health crisis, an economic crisis, a political crisis, a racial crisis, and a climate crisis, all of which were connected to the pandemic and came together in an unprecedented way.

Many people shared the outrage that Bowleg and Krieger expressed about the fact that the burden of the pandemic was unequally distributed. The surveillance system that would have helped document these inequities and devise precise and targeted interventions was not in place.

The Elusive Dashboard

An accurate data dashboard is essential for the Public Health Approach. In chapter 2, I documented how population thinking was discovered thanks to the London Bills of Mortality, a "dashboard" of the causes of death over several decades. Their equivalent would be a system that provides information about how the prevalence of infection progresses across place and time. When governments have such dashboards, they can devise precise interventions, especially in terms of consequential decisions for the future of children, such as school closures, or for the economy, such as business closures.

Fortunately, the US surveillance system has reacted quickly to the shock wave of COVID-19. The December 2021 issue of the *American Journal of Public Health* was dedicated to the impact of COVID-19 on surveillance and surveys in the United States. Denys T. Lau, Nabarun Dasgupta, Hua He, and Paulina Sosa reviewed the current US surveillance system and ways to prepare and respond effectively to the COVID-19 pandemic and to future emergencies.[27] When the COVID-19 pandemic began, the United States had a fragmented system that collected information in person and that lacked modern electronic techniques for processing this data. The set of reports in the December 2021 special issue showed that, collectively, federal, state, and city surveillance and survey programs began to remedy the defective structures, and improved plans to collect, process, and disseminate information.

However, despite expert knowledge and good intentions, the United States is still missing the information that formed the core of the 1918 Public Health Service survey: estimates of incidence and fatality rates and comparisons of these data across time, people, and places. The United States needs a modern health monitoring system that collects, analyzes, and disseminates data about infection, hospitalization, and fatality rates in real time. Surveys like the 1918 Public Health Service remain indispensable for reliable estimates about pandemic diseases. Such surveys are feasible, and modern infrastructure provides the optimal conditions for performing them. Examples include, in the United Kingdom, the REal-time Assessment of Community Transmission (REACT) of SARS-CoV-2 virus, and the Office for National Statistics COVID-19 infection survey.[28] Spain's seroepidemiological survey of SARS-CoV-2 virus infection ("Encuesta Seroepidemiológica de la Infección por el Virus SARS-CoV-2 en España; ENE-COVID") is another outstanding example of what every government should have done.[29] The survey was nationwide, although it excluded care-home residents, hospitalized people, people in prisons, nuns and friars in convents, and residents in other collective facilities. As in the 1918 US Public Health Service survey, researchers using two-stage sampling selected 35,883 households across Spanish provinces, cities, and municipalities. Households were randomly sampled. All residents in the household were invited to participate. The final sample included 102,562 individuals of all ages. This study relied on the Spanish National Health System. Serum specimens were collected from all participants two to four weeks apart. The results were surprising. The national prevalence of infection was only 5%. It was higher in the capital, Madrid (10%) and lower in coastal areas (<3%). An important observation was that around one-third of seropositive participants was asymptomatic.

The Spanish survey is exemplary. Preparing for future pandemics requires a vibrant health monitoring system—a better term than the commonly used "surveillance system"—that is granular enough to track their progression in communities that traditionally are hurt the most. While modernizing the public-health data infrastructure of the US federal government and 3,050 state and local health departments will cost a lot, the future of the Public Health Approach depends on it.[30]

The Public Health Approach

The Public Health Approach has contributed to understanding some determinants of human health and to devising policies to control them. An immense number of human lives have been either or both healthier and longer than if the Public Health Approach had not been implemented. A sequel to the scientific revolution, the Public Health Approach began when population thinking was first applied to data collected in London to track the epidemics of bubonic plague in the seventeenth century. This shift in perspective led to major changes in how scientists, doctors, and researchers think about and study public health, a few of which were mentioned in this book. For instance, in the eighteenth century, comparing groups provided the scientific support for smallpox inoculation as an effective strategy for preventing people from dying from or experiencing a severe case of the disease. In the nineteenth century, sanitary reforms that were later supported by bacteriology dramatically reduced the burden of endemic infectious diseases in urban centers. In the twentieth century, evidence from a population-based cohort study debunked the eugenicist argument that tuberculosis was inherited, revealing instead the role of social determinants; a randomized controlled trial in 1947 showed that streptomycin was an effective treatment for pulmonary tuberculosis; and new population-based causal inference determined the effects of consuming tobacco on both lung cancer and cardiovascular disease, resulting in public health campaigns that inverted the trends of tobacco consumptions in many populations. Statistical methods handling a study sample as a supraindividual were used to assess the efficacy of treatment for HIV/AIDS. Population thinking applied to police violence, incarceration, and deaths of despair revealed patterns that indicated structural causes that can be studied and changed.

However, the lessons that this book covers were learned at a very high human cost for public health and society: many more illnesses could have been prevented and many more lives could have been saved in the process of establishing the foundations of the Public Health Approach. What we have learned is that a change in perspective from individual medical care to strategies for protecting the health of entire populations is not sufficient for an effective Public Health Approach. This epilogue reviews the four elements required for a Public Health Approach to produce the desired results. First, population thinking needs to be based in science. Second, it needs to be all-inclusive; any type of thinking that discriminates against some sectors of the population based on their culture, ethnicity, nationality, or sexuality is incompatible with the Public Health Approach. Third, the implementation of the public health consequences needs to be just; that is, it needs to avoid harmful discrimination. Fourth, it needs to be participatory, by which I mean that it needs integrate the input of the public and participate in democratic discourse.

Science-Based, All-Inclusive, Just, and Participatory

Science-Based

Theories that have been tested scientifically are essential for devising effective interventions that can be implemented safely among a very large number of people. Relying on science also means rigorously establishing what is the cause of an illness and rejecting the widespread tendency to arrive at conclusions about causality based on observations of individual people.

Solid scientific bases offer safeguards for public health interventions. When a doctor hurts an individual patient with an inappropriate treatment, it is malpractice. A doctor usually makes mistakes one patient at a time. Public health interventions occur at a different scale that can include millions of people. Even a small risk of an unwanted effect at that scale can translate into large numbers of injured or harmed individuals.

Consider the potential side effects of the COVID-19 vaccines. In the spring of 2021, it was reported that in a group of around 20 million people who had received the AstraZeneca vaccine in the United Kingdom and European Union countries, twenty-five experienced serious blood clots and nine of those twenty-five died. The potential mortality risk was extremely small ($9/20,000,000$), but the target population of COVID-19 vaccines is several hundred times larger than 20 million.[1] A small risk can have mass consequences. For the 300 million Americans there could be 135 cases if the risk applied similarly to every age group. The distribution of the vaccine was stopped until it was shown that the population benefits of the vaccine outweighed the risk.

The science-based dimension of the Public Health Approach distinguishes it from any other organized intervention regarding health. Interventions that lack scientific foundations have resulted in actions that were often ineffective and sometimes counterproductive. In antiquity, for instance, governments invested in public works that removed sewage and provided clean water. Cities required garbage removal, pipes, and roads. These public works improved the quality of life for urban residents, but the link between these measures and the endemic dysentery or other gastrointestinal diseases could not be established without a population-based science. Keeping cities clean benefited their inhabitants, but in some cases, when contaminated sewage was washed away into the waters of rivers and lakes that were used for drinking and cooking and for washing people, clothes, and bed linens, these public health interventions could paradoxically sustain endemic diseases and amplify epidemics of gastrointestinal diseases.

During the Middle Ages, urban magistrates, unaware that plague could be transmitted by fleas on rats, attempted to control epidemics by sealing plague victims and their relatives in their homes until they eventually died. These actions were mostly ineffective because the rats and the fleas they carried could escape from houses where people were sick and infect households whose inhabitants were still healthy. Magistrates turned to killing cats and dogs, which they viewed as potential carriers of the disease to neighboring houses. However, these animals killed rats and thus kept their fleas away from humans. This was policing, not public health. These interventions were not based on a scientific understanding of the cause of a disease.

The sanitary reformers of the nineteenth century offer an example of the dire consequences of not basing public health policies on science. They understood that prevention was the preferred strategy and focused on building healthy environments in expanding industrial cities. Although these policies decreased the rates of endemic infectious diseases in cities, the speculative nature of the theories on which they based their policies betrayed them. The fear of invisible miasmas was enough to justify a consensus around sanitary laws, but policies based on the belief that miasmas caused disease could not control extraordinary epidemics. A legacy was tarnished in a few years after the cholera epidemic of 1892 which was a debacle in sanitarian Hamburg, but not in contagionist Altona

All-Inclusive

Public health officials identify collective threats against which we cannot protect ourselves individually and devise safe collective responses. The success of those responses depends on reaching everyone. They must be all-inclusive. This is as true for vaccines as it is for environmental protection or occupational safety. Viruses, air pollution, and occupational risks are universal threats. Equitable access is what makes public health interventions effective. The principle of all-inclusiveness is encapsulated in the concept of a population strategy of prevention instead of the medical focus on individuals who are at a high risk of contracting a specific disease.

The enforcement powers of public health officials contribute to the all-inclusive nature of their policies. They can also be used to prevent a minority from jeopardizing the common good. Refusing to comply with public health measures because of personal preference, as vaccine refusers do, defeats the goals of public health policies. In 1905, in *Jacobson v. Massachusetts*, seven of the nine US Supreme Court justices agreed that mandatory vaccinations were constitutional.[2] Justice John Marshall Harlan explained their reasoning:

> The liberty secured by the Constitution of the United States does not import an absolute right in each person to be at all times, and in all circumstances, wholly freed from restraint, nor is it an element in such liberty that one person, or a minority of persons residing in any community and enjoying the benefits of its local government, should have power to dominate the majority when supported in their action by the authority of the State. It is within the police power of a State to enact a compulsory vaccination law, and

it is for the legislature, and not for the courts, to determine in the first instance whether vaccination is or is not the best mode for the prevention of smallpox and the protection of the public health.[3]

James Colgrove and Ronald Bayer,[4] Lawrence O. Gostin,[5] and Wendy K. Mariner and colleagues[6] have noted that the context in 1905 was different from that of today. In 1905, the Court's decision in *Jacobson v. Massachusetts* could be invoked to justify eugenicist sterilization and coercive measures that targeted powerless citizens, such as the quarantining of prostitutes during World War I to prevent the spread of syphilis. Still, this decision articulated a key value that the freedom of the individual must sometimes be subordinated to the interest of the common welfare. This is the concept that helped introduce policies regarding mandatory childhood vaccines and protection against tobacco smoke in public places.[7]

The principle of all-inclusiveness also explains why public health has historically been incompatible with authoritarian regimes or ideologies of the radical right. Those ideologies exclude part of the population for arbitrary reasons. Far-right authoritarian governments usually promote chauvinistic, racist, or xenophobic policies that limit the access of immigrants and what they define as "deviant" minorities to public health measures. Viruses do not respect borders, religious beliefs, sexual identities, or social classes. Environmental pollution is not limited to certain neighborhoods. Any artificial limits on what defines a population hamper the goals of public health.

Just

Examples abound of uncontrolled public health practices that led to tragedies. The Tuskegee Syphilis Study, conducted by the US Public Health Service, lasted for four decades, from 1932 to 1972.[8] It involved 399 infected Black men and 201 controls. Many of the participants were low-income, rural sharecroppers from Macon County, Alabama. By 1947, penicillin was a widely available and effective treatment for syphilis, but participants in the Tuskegee study were not treated or informed that they could receive medical care elsewhere. As Vanessa Gamble notes, the Tuskegee study has come to "symbolize racism in medicine, misconduct in human research, the arrogance of physicians, and government abuse of Black people."[9] It added offense to an already long series of medical abuses.

Other examples of unjust public health practices include the studies run in the 1940s by United States Public Health Service investigators in Guatemala that involved over 5,000 people, many of them infected with bacteria that cause sexually transmitted diseases without their consent[10] and the widely accepted belief among public health officials of the early twentieth century that disabilities were hereditary determinants of health. The latter belief led to the sterilization of people with disabilities or the killing of disabled infants at birth in the name of eugenics. Between 1919 and 1979 the State of California ordered approximately 20,000 nonconsensual sterilizations for eugenic purposes, representing one third of the more than 60,000 such procedures in the United States in the twentieth century.[11] Another example of the abuse of public health policies is how Los Angeles public health officials participated in efforts to restrict the number of Mexican immigrants through the 1920s and to expel Mexicans and Filipinos in the 1930s.[12]

Sadly, there are many other incidents of xenophobic or discriminatory applications of public health policies, especially in the first half of the twentieth century. As historian Susan Reverby has noted, "These practices happen to communities, not just to the actual individuals. The trust of public health officials is eroded when knowledge, especially of overwrought or false information, circulates and becomes the symbol for mistrust even when details of what happened are unknown."[13] Theories that interrogate, expose, and challenge assumptions about power and privilege such as intersectionality,[14] emphasize how important justice is in the field of public health.[15]

Participatory

Public health policies work better when they are implemented by the people.[16] No top-down process will both reach everyone in the population and generate trust in the government. Grassroots organizations have often played key roles in shaping policies to control epidemics. These include front-line LGBTQ organizations;[17] organizations of Black women[18] or workers,[19] and faith-based organizations[20] that have encouraged their members to participate in public health measures in hard-to-reach communities.

In their introduction to a special issue of the *American Journal of Public Health* that marked the fiftieth anniversary of the Stonewall riots, Stewart Landers and Farzana Kapadia noted that during the HIV/AIDS epidemic, the LGBTQ community embraced the principle of "nothing about us, without us."[21] The AIDS crisis would have been less severe if health care services for people with AIDS had been less underfunded and if government public health officials had been more willing to meet the needs of the LGBTQ population.[22] The activism of the LGBTQ community during the first decades of the AIDS epidemic gathered momentum that led to significant changes to national law. As psychologist Perry Halkitis has noted, "without Stonewall we have no AIDS activism, and without AIDS activism we have no marriage equality—a social condition that surely has had a beneficial effect on our health."[23]

In 2010, President Barack Obama signed into law the National HIV/AIDS Strategy, a five-year plan for reducing infections, improving care and outcomes for people living with HIV, and reducing HIV-related disparities. The strategy did not include sexual and reproductive health rights or gender-based violence, leading women's organizations, particularly those of Black and Brown women, to request it. All these grassroots movements inspire and contribute to the success of others, a point Dázon Dixon Diallo has made:

> Over the course of history, Black women have shown that when we organize to change things for ourselves, we change things for everyone. Recent and historical events have shaped this truth as the evidence—civil and voting rights, sexual harassment accountability, gender-based violence, housing and food justice, environmental justice, economic justice, human rights, racial and reproductive justice, science and technology, education equity, civic and political engagement, abolitionism, ending state violence against Black and Brown communities, and fighting concurrent pandemics.[24]

Grassroots movements have also been effective around these issues in the workplace. Coalitions or centers for occupational safety and health emerged in the 1970s as decentralized organizations that required input from workers, including their knowledge of work processes, in the design of workplaces. Frequently these organizations have "committees composed of local health and safety professionals, technicians, and activists who help union locals in obtaining information about occupational hazards, conduct educational sessions for interested workers, and prepare brief, educational pamphlets on specific health and safety hazards."[25]

Faith-based organizations have built vast coalitions that promote immunization in at-risk and underserved populations, establish sanctuaries for threatened migrants, and contain the Ebola virus and HIV in hard-to-reach communities.[26]

Some well-intentioned public health policies have failed because key stakeholders were not involved. In 2012, the New York City Department of Health and Mental Hygiene attempted to ban the sale of "sugary beverages" that were sold in containers larger than sixteen ounces in restaurants, in stadiums, in movie theaters, and at mobile food vending vehicles in New York City. Failure to comply could have led to a $200 fine. This science-based policy was designed to prevent obesity. Christina A. Roberto and Jennifer L. Pomeranz, who have reviewed 38,701 documents containing arguments and oral testimony about the proposed policy, found that 47% favored the restriction and 50% opposed it. Those in favor argued that obesity is a major public health problem, that highly sugared drinks are the greatest contributors to obesity, that portion sizes are too large, and that the government has a responsibility to protect the health of the public. The group that was in favor of the proposed law consisted largely of doctors and other health care professionals (54%) and members of the general public (36%).[27]

Those who opposed the proposed law consisted mostly of members of the public (57%) and owners of businesses that sold soft drinks (18%). This group argued that sugary beverages weren't addictive like tobacco and thus weren't an appropriate target for government intervention, that the policy was an example of government intrusion on freedoms, that there wasn't any evidence that the policy would change consumer behavior or reduce obesity, and that the policy would hurt businesses unfairly. These arguments won the day. Two lower courts ruled against the proposed law and a New York State appeals court struck it down. State Supreme Court Justice Milton A. Tingling Jr. ruled that the ban's loopholes, for example a lack of a ban on refills, "defeat[ed] and/or serve[d] to gut the purpose of the rule." Marion Nestle, who tells the complex story in *Soda Politics*,[28] suggests that the outcome might have been different if a text of the law had been developed with the active involvement of the communities it would have most impacted. Ben Jealous, president of the chapter of the National Association for the Advancement of Colored People that filed a brief opposing the ban, said that although his group would support the idea of a ban, "you have to do it well. . . . It's not the details about the policy. This is about organizing. This is about come talk to us, right? Let's figure out how to do this together."[29]

Who Are the Switchers?

Not everyone agrees with all the public health recommendations all the time, but the ideological composition of camps that support or oppose policies vary according to the historical context. When Boston clergy urged doctors to immunize the population using variolation in 1721, doctors were opposed. In the nineteenth century, sanitary movement reformers were opposed to the policies that laboratory scientists urged: mandating quarantines and shutting down businesses during pandemics of cholera.

People who hesitate to follow public health guidance usually believe that their decisions impact only themselves. They often feel that whether they will contract a disease depends on factors that elude human decisions or action and population-level calculations of risk are meaningless. Whether they will be victims of COVID-19 is only a question of chance, or if their faith tells them so, of Providence: their fate is independent of that of others. They are highly influenced by isolated or even fictitious anecdotes that support their skepticism. They do not perceive that by refusing the public health recommendation they endanger the whole population.

In contrast, people who follow public health recommendations perceive that it is the optimal course of action for them as individuals and for their population collectively. They are acting, from a science perspective, in their own best interest since it will represent the path of lower risk of harm to them and others too. They believe that it is only as a collective that we can learn about ourselves, identify collective threats, and devise collective responses. They understand that even though no outcome is guaranteed, the most likely outcome is that people who are vaccinated are less likely to be infected, to get seriously ill, and if they do get ill, to die from COVID-19. This may be the main motivation for those who comply with public health recommendations, but some certainly realize that the collective vaccination will shorten the duration of the epidemic, save small businesses from bankruptcy, reduce the education deficit in children, and prevent overcrowding in hospitals and deaths from COVID-19.

Modernizing Public Health

Amid the evidence of progress in public health, there is a major source of concern: a dramatic decrease in the number of people working in the field of public health. Katie Sellers and colleagues, who have analyzed a nationally representative survey conducted in 2017 of professionals employed by federal, state, and local governments in the field of public health, note that a very high percentage of respondees planned to retire within the next few years and another large proportion planned to leave the field before retirement age.[30] These departures mean a tremendous loss of experience and knowledge for the field.

During the COVID-19 pandemic, there was increasing violence against public health officials at the hands of vaccine refusers. Julie A. Ward, Elizabeth M. Stone, Paulani Mui, and Beth Resnick reported in the *American Journal of Public Health* that from March 2020 to January 2021, employees in local health departments in the United States reported at least 1,499 incidents of harassment; public health officials experienced "structural and political undermining of their professional duties, marginalization of their expertise, social villainization, and disillusionment." A third of the position departures were linked to this violence.[31]

These despicable behaviors did not prevent the implementation of the COVID-19 vaccination campaign. Hundreds of millions voted with their arms. The violence that some expressed against public health officials should not hide the fact that the COVID-19 response has succeeded better than most previous public health campaigns in the United States. Thomas Quade, who was health commissioner for Geauga County, Ohio, noted that "while we did experience a tremendous amount of antagonism, we also got thank-you cards almost every day. We got people bringing us boxes of cookies for staff."[32]

This demonstration of effectiveness opens up vast new potential for the field of public health. Indeed, while some professionals appear to be moving away from the field, among younger generations, there is growing interest in being exposed to public health in college. Paul C. Erwin and his coauthors have called attention to the increase in the number of bachelor's degrees in public health conferred in the United States over the last three decades: from 750 in 1992 to 6,500 in 2012 to 13,000 in 2016.[33] These stem from efforts of the Association of Schools and Programs of Public Health to increase the number of undergraduate programs in public health education and the inclusion of undergraduate degree programs in the accreditation standards of the Council on Education for Public Health. In 2021, the council's website listed 209 accredited bachelor's degree programs.[34] These degree programs are offered in a variety of institutional settings, from those with both accredited undergraduate and graduate degree programs to those with only an undergraduate program. They offer a unique window of opportunity to teach the Public Health Approach to a greater number of future professionals. The wave of undergraduate degrees will not replace graduate degrees like the master of public health as a means to a career in the field, they but increase the familiarity with public health of a new generation of lawyers, doctors, engineers, and so on. Hopefully this book will be used to teach the Public Health Approach to undergraduate students.

The challenge is to entice people with undergraduate degrees in public health to become public health professionals. Offering competitive salaries, conveying a sense of mission, and providing space for creativity and new initiatives will help employers in the field of public health keep their workforces vibrant. Maybe even more importantly, public health requires to be modernized.

We have inherited an aberrant system in which expensive health care, often in emergency care units, is the first level of response to health issues.[35] Because medical care is the main interface people have with the health sector, they do not experience the fact that medicine is an individual response to an individual health problem, whereas public health is a collective response to a collective threat. Enforcing medical decisions is unjust, but not enforcing public health policies leads to injustice. A modern health sector requires greater investments into prevention and population approaches to health. The resources exist. Estimates of the value of wasteful spending on medical care in the United States range from $600 billion to more than $1.9 trillion per year, or roughly $1,800 to $5,700 per person per year.[36] This wasteful spending can be avoided and the resources can be used differently.

In many ways the current social and public health challenges are as large as those the sanitary reformers faced in the nineteenth century. We face a major environmental threat, severe inequities, mass uprooting and migrations from poorer to richer regions of the world, and a growing focus on the way social determinants can induce ill health. However, twenty-first-century public health professionals have a tool that those in the nineteenth century lacked: the modern Public Health Approach.

For the first six months of the SARS-CoV-2 pandemic, January to June 2020, the US press used the terms "epidemiology" and "public health" up to 100 times more often than they had during the same period in 2019.[37] However, a greater use of the term "public health" does not mean that it is understood. Allow me to repeat this. It may still not be common knowledge that medicine and public health have different approaches to health. Doctors give prescriptions to individuals who are free to comply with them or not, but a public health recommendation is a collective response to a collective threat. For the policy to be effective, everyone in the population must know about it and have access to its benefits. That kind of response is needed in order to protect the water we drink and cook with and the air we breathe, to protect children from being exploited as workers, or to control a devastating epidemic using vaccines. Individually, we are powerless against these scourges.

The time is ripe for explaining how public health thinks. During the COVID-19 pandemic, the majority of the US population complied with public health recommendations regarding quarantine, masks, physical distancing, and vaccination. This may mark a watershed moment between the time when the Public Health Approach was understood only by scientists in population sciences and a future time when every resident of the United States and elsewhere integrates public health ideas and recommendations into their daily life.

There are reasons to be optimistic about the short-term future. A mental shift from individual to population thinking is not enough in itself, but it can make a difference. It is my hope that this book will contribute to a wider understanding of the principles and scientific underpinnings of the Public Health Approach.

Acknowledgments

After serving as the editor-in-chief of the *American Journal of Public Health* for seven years and processing 30,000 submissions, I became convinced that the Public Health Approach is insufficiently understood by the public at large and that I had the expertise to help remedy this situation. My expertise as a historian is in the history of scientific methods used to study populations—that is, methods in which counts and statistics play an important role—and the search for causes in those contexts. My previous books, *A History of Epidemiologic Methods and Concepts* (Basel: Birkhäuser Basel, 2004) and *Enigmas of Health and Disease: How Epidemiology Helps Unravel Scientific Mysteries* (New York: Columbia University Press, 2014), focused on the evolution of epidemiology. This book is about the methods and concepts used in the field of public health, which is a broader topic than epidemiology.

Matthew McAdam, my editor at Johns Hopkins University Press, has played a major role in shaping this short book around the simple message that the Public Health Approach is built on a shift in perspective from the individual to the population. Matt's vision inspired me. The draft has been edited for content and style by Michael C. Costanza, Theodore Brown, Mark Rothstein, Dan Fox, Charles Dibble, and copyeditor Kate Babbitt. They were merciless in their comments and helped shape the final version.

I am deeply grateful to Kristin Heitman for her comments on chapter 2, to Henry Blackburn for his comments on chapter 6, and to Sonja Swanson for her comments on chapter 7 and for drawing the graph that appears in that chapter.

Becoming a part of the American Public Health Association (APHA) has been another source of education and knowledge. The 150-year-old association has a dense network of connections with professionals in the field from the local to the federal level and is widely respected for its unique role in the defense and promotion of public health.

I am grateful to Georges Benjamin, executive director of the APHA, for entrusting the leadership of the *American Journal of Public Health* to me. Dr. Benjamin, who is regularly cited as one of the most influential persons in medicine, is even more influential in public health. His tremendous knowledge of the people and issues connected with public health has given me insight into the field and into the readership of the journal in the monthly meetings that we hold. I am also indebted to my colleagues on the journal's production team, in particular to its leader, Brian Selzer, the Deputy Director of Publication Services.

My editorial assistants were students through 2022. They were, in chronological order, Olufunmilayo Makinde (University of Maryland), Shreya Patel (George Washington University), Marwa Fadlalla (University of Memphis School of Public Health), Paulina Sosa (Johns Hopkins University), and Shokhari Tate (George Washington University).

The editorial team of the *American Journal of Public Health* consists of outstanding researchers and public health people who have been guiding me about the topics I choose each month and about key editorial decisions that we made at the changes of US federal administrations and when the COVID-19 pandemic broke out. The Student Think Tank, a group of six dynamic students that is renewed every year, has made sure that the perspective of the new generation of public health people is present in the journal. David Sundwal, former executive director of the Utah Department of Health, has helped build a multipartisan group of former health officers of states and territories. They have been advising me as editor since 2017. I owe them a broader vision and understanding of public health.

The historical perspective of the book comes from years of studying the history of the methods and concepts of epidemiology. The National Library of Medicine (grant G13 LM010884-02) funded the research for this book. I am indebted for their expertise on the history of epidemiological methods to my colleagues Henry Blackburn, Kristin Heitman, Anne Hardy, and Jan Vandenbroucke.

I am grateful to my colleagues at the Barry Commoner Center for Health and the Environment, and its director, Steven Markowitz, for giving me the opportunity to teach the content of this book at Queens College, City University of New York. Special thanks to Christiana Oyewande, who was the teaching assistant for the first version in the spring semester of 2022.

My family, Sophie, Léon, and Bob, are great supporters, and I hope they will like the book. The book is dedicated to my mother, Linda. It became a topic of discussion in the daily calls we had during the pandemic. She read several drafts, and I worked on her comments until she said she liked the book. This book is with her and for her.

Appendix

How Old Is the Public Health Approach?

Historians usually find the roots of public health in the earliest human societies and distinguish its premodern from its modern manifestations. The transition took place in the seventeenth century.[1]

Before the seventeenth century, most, if not all, medical frameworks were centered on the individual, including those of the physicians of ancient Greece, of traditional Chinese medicine, or of Aztec medicine.[2] The medical models and treatment techniques differed between the regional systems in Europe, Asia, or America, but they all considered health as resulting from an equilibrium, first within the individual and then between the individual and the global environment. Physicians believed that many factors could create an imbalance in the human organism that resulted in disease. Since these factors varied according to the individual's temperament, the seasons, the astrological setting, and the weather, the explanations doctors gave for why health was lost were different for each person. Because every individual deserved a specific diagnosis, a specific prognosis, and treatment tailored to that person's needs, doctors usually did not see health as a community issue. That is why counting patients was not routine in premodern health care systems.

Had death counts been available before the seventeenth century, population thinking might have become important then. In the absence of health statistics, health practitioners or policymakers could only have intuited the population dimension of health. This appendix explores whether there was some intuition of population thinking in antiquity and the Middle Ages.

Epidemics

Epidemics have an obvious population dimension and are therefore a good point to start exploring traces of the Public Health Approach in the past. Epidemic comes from the ancient Greek *epi*, which means "upon," and *demos*, "population." An epidemic is an event that suddenly affects many people. It is unclear when the first epidemic occurred. Both the invention of writing and the first recorded epidemic are from the same time and place, about 4,000 years ago in Mesopotamia, a valley between two rivers, the Tigris and the Euphrates.[3] Four thousand years ago, it was the site of large urban civilizations.

In *Plagues and Peoples*, historian William McNeill posits that the set of circumstances necessary for an infectious epidemic to take place occurred for the first time in Mesopotamia.[4] A first condition was that humans shared dwellings with large domestic animals. Most of the bacteria, parasites, and viruses responsible for historical epidemics and pandemics appear to have crossed from the animal kingdom to the human species. Cows, buffalos, pigs, and horses were immune to these microorganisms because of natural selection, but they were new organisms for the human body. Living with large, domesticated animals created the conditions for their parasites to cross the species barrier and cause measles, mumps, tuberculosis, smallpox, and other infectious diseases in humans.

For each index human case to spread and evolve into an epidemic, a microorganism needs to constantly find susceptible people to infect, multiply itself, and continue its cycle. McNeill relied on a simulation that indicated that a population had to have 300,000 to 400,000 persons to provide enough hosts for a microorganism to cause an epidemic.[5] This was met in the network of Sumerian cities of Mesopotamia. The earliest descriptions of a lethal epidemic are from the Epic of Gilgamesh, a Babylonian text, and in a pharaonic text from Egypt, both from about 4,000 years ago.

There is no historical evidence of an effective, concerted human effort to control epidemics when they first occurred and throughout antiquity and the Middle Ages. Our best source of information comes from a catalogue of epidemics in the Chinese Empire that appears in an appendix to *Plagues and Peoples*.[6] In China, during the last Empire (243 BCE to 1911 CE), the number of epidemics increased exponentially.[7] The Chinese Empire appears to have been powerless against epidemics. This must have been true for other civilizations then, even though there are no data to document this conjecture. After 2000 BCE, other large networks of cities developed over millennia. Many became interconnected by commercial routes that connected Asia to Europe. After the fifteenth century, trade routes connected Europe and the Americas and finally the whole human world.[8] The interconnectedness of human societies has contributed to the emergence of pandemics such as cholera, flu, HIV/AIDS, and SARS-CoV-2/COVID-19.

Epidemics seem to have evolved without any public health obstacle until at least the seventeenth century. Effective control of the epidemics would have required a Public Health Approach, and there was none. This suggests that the perspective shift from individual thinking about health to population thinking did not occur before the seventeenth century.

Precursors to Population Thinking

Documents from antiquity and the Middle Ages can be used to assess when the intellectual tools for analyzing epidemics and forming appropriate public health policy interventions emerged. I have found nine documents indicating traces of population thinking prior to the seventeenth century (table A.1). They can be categorized into three types: spiritual, medical, and administrative. Approaching these texts is not straightforward. There are considerable concerns about their authenticity and the accuracy of the translations. Some were originally written in ancient languages and then translated. For example, we do not have the original Hippocratic treatises written in Greek. We work with translations of these texts into Latin or Arabic that were retranslated into Greek and later into English. Ulpian and Petrarch wrote in Latin, and al-Rāzī wrote in ancient Arabic. Having myself attempted to translate some of

Historical documents suggestive of population thinking before the seventeenth century

TYPE	DOCUMENT	CENTURIES	TOPIC
Spiritual	Old Testament Book of Samuel	10th century BCE	King David's census (Israel)
Spiritual	Old Testament Book of Daniel	6th to 2nd centuries BCE	Captivity of Israelites in Babylonia
Medical notes	Medical notes of Hippocrates	5th century BCE	Air, waters, and places (Greece)
Medical notes	Medical notes of Hippocrates	5th century BCE	Epidemic of mumps (Greece)
Administrative	Ulpian	3rd century CE	Estates and heritage (Rome)
Medical notes	al-Rāzī	9th to 10th centuries CE	Clinical study (Persia)
Administrative	Plague rolls	15th to 17th centuries CE	Quarantine (Europe)
Medical notes	Petrarch	15th to 16th centuries CE	Evaluation of medical expertise (Italy)
Medical notes	Bartolomé Hidalgo de Agüero	16th century CE	Treatment of wounds (Spain)

these texts from Latin and Greek, I am very much aware of the amount of interpretation that goes into the process. Reading several translations is recommended to get a sense of what their authors were saying. In this chapter, I am not placing quotation marks when I provide my own adaptation of the original text, but I provide a link to an available translation.[9] Nonetheless, these texts document the mode of thinking of major intellectuals of their times. This appendix discusses all of them except two that required too much background: the Book of Samuel from the Old Testament[10] and a document written by Ulpian, also known as Gnaeus Domitius Annius Ulpianus (ca. 170–223 CE), which suggests that the amount of an annuity derived from an inherited property should relate to the age of the beneficiary.[11]

Mumps in Thasos, 500 BCE

A 2,000-year-old document included in table A.1 describes an epidemic characterized by swelling of the face and testicles and a dry cough. The location was the small Greek island of Thasos located in the upper north of the Aegean Sea. The author noted that swellings appeared about the ears, in many on either side, and in the greatest number on both sides, without a fever that would confine the patient to bed; in all cases swellings disappeared without giving trouble, neither did any of them come to suppuration, as is common in swellings from other causes. The swellings were of a lax, large, diffused character, without inflammation or pain, and went away without any critical sign. The swellings seized children, adults, and mostly those who engaged in exercises at the palestra and gymnasium. The swellings seldom attacked women. Many patients had dry coughs without expectoration, without voice hoarseness. In some instances, earlier, and in others later, inflammations seized one and sometimes both testicles. Some of these cases had fever and some had not.[12]

The note is typical for the Hippocratic school of physicians that is referred to as the Hippocratic Collection.[13] These doctors lived in ancient Greece and nearby regions about 500 years before the common era. Their work has considerably influenced Western medicine, from the description of clinical signs (e.g., the Hippocratic facies) to medical ethics (e.g., the Hippocratic oath). These texts do not include prayers or magical incantations because these doctors did not invoke supernatural forces in their practice. The accuracy of the clinical description of the epidemic in Thasos is such that any modern clinician would immediately recognize mumps, but 2,500 years ago, these symptoms were not considered to be evidence of a specific disease. The novel epidemic affected both children and adults. Only a few people were already immune to it, as was the case for SARS-CoV-2/COVID-19 in 2020.[14] Today we know that mumps is a viral disease that spreads through direct contact with saliva or respiratory droplets from the mouth, nose, or throat of an infected person. The text mentions that men who visited gyms and stadiums were commonly affected.

As is typical for the Hippocratic treatises, the author never mentioned counting patients and their symptoms. The Greek physician began by noting that in "many" people, swellings appeared at the ears on one side only and in "the greatest number" on both sides. "None," "some," "few," "most," "all," are all expressions of frequency in the Hippocratic texts, but they are not precise. This is a reliable indication that the number of cases were estimated and not counted. Had doctors gone through the time-consuming process of recording cases, categorizing them, and summing them across categories to compare them, they most likely would have reported exact numbers.

But don't these texts indicate a qualitative form of population thinking? Aren't "none," "some," "few," "most," and "all" legitimate ways of conveying the frequency of events? Yes and no. The text quoted above undoubtedly conveys a sense of perceived frequency. Most "patients" had the bilateral inflammation of the sublingual glands (aka parotitis) that is responsible for the typical facial swelling of mumps. The doctor also says that patients had a painful inflammation of "sometimes" one and "sometimes" both testicles,[15] what is known today as epididymo-orchitis. This information is vague, however.

Why didn't the doctor who wrote this text count his patients? He belonged to the Hippocratic doctors, a school of traveling doctors. They would pitch their tent on the marketplace, and patients would line up. Hippocratic doctors kept detailed notes of their observations. The Hippocratic Collection includes dozens of individual clinical histories. It would have been feasible for them to count the number of patients and number of symptoms and provide exact proportions of those who had bilateral inflammation of the sublingual glands, for example.

Hippocratic doctors most likely did not count their patients because they did not expect that the effort of adding, subtracting, and dividing would provide them with knowledge that would improve their medical practice. Note that the physician only describes signs and symptoms. He never refers to them as a disease. Mumps is a modern name for this particular group of symptoms. The description does not suggest that the patients are suffering from the same disease. They are individuals having similar symptoms. They are not "cases" of mumps. In 500 BCE, there was no conceptual basis for saying that 60%–70% of mumps "cases" were symptomatic or that parotitis generally occurs in 95% of pediatric "cases" or that epididymo-orchitis occurs in 5% to 10% of all the symptomatic "cases."

The medical writer of the texts in the Hippocratic Collection believed that diseases that affected many people simultaneously, such as the mumps epidemic in Thasos, were caused by a form of air pollution. Miasmas caused by invisible but smelly particles that floated in the air affected susceptible people who inhaled the bad air.[16] Miasma comes from the Greek word μίασμα, which can be translated as "pollution."[17] For the Hippocratic doctors, when many people were seized simultaneously by the same symptoms, miasmas were the cause.[18]

Doctors did not feel comfortable in these situations. Medicine was about treating individuals who required individualized prescriptions. Because medical knowledge and skills were ineffective against the effects of miasmas, doctors were released from their duty to provide care in such cases. Instead, they advised people to breathe superficially and escape as soon as possible from areas where miasmas occurred.[19]

In antiquity, medical knowledge was inadequate for responding to these mass phenomena because their causes and control can be understood only at the population level, a perspective that did not exist then. Hippocratic medicine was primarily medical care for the individual.

Airs, Waters, and Places
The ideas developed at the beginning of a treatise titled *Airs, Waters, and Places* seem very modern. The medical writer indicates that whoever wishes to investigate medicine properly, should proceed as follows: first, consider the seasons of the year, and the effects each of them produces, for they are not at all alike. Second, the hot and cold winds, especially those common to all countries, and then those specific to each locality. Third, one must also consider the qualities of the waters, which differ in taste and weight. Similarly, when one comes into a city as a stranger, the newcomer ought to consider its situation, how it is exposed to the winds and the rising of the sun. The influence of the sun is not the same

whether the city lies to the north, to the south, to the rising or to the setting sun. These elements should be considered most attentively, as well as whether the waters the inhabitants use, are marshy and soft, or hard, running from elevated and rocky situations, and whether they are saltish and unfit for cooking. The ground, whether it be naked and deficient in water, or wooded and well-watered, and whether it lies in a hollow, confined situation, or is elevated and cold. The mode in which the inhabitants live, and what are their pursuits, whether they are fond of drinking and eating to excess, given to indolence, or are fond of exercise and labor, and don't eat and drink in excess.[20]

To a modern reader, it seems like the Hippocratic doctor is listing environmental risk factors related to winds and the quality of the water and the soil. However, this doctor did not make a one-to-one association with specific environmental conditions and specific diseases. He does not view the wind, the waters, the soil, or the air as an individual cause of disease. That kind of thinking did not exist five hundred years before the common era. The author of this text considered airs, waters, and places together as one complex environment that might be associated with the symptoms of individual people. This holistic reasoning locates the individual in the center of a complex interaction between the environment and the individual's inner constitution, which included their character or temperament (e.g., bilious or phlegmatic) their diet, heredity, and so on. This is more obvious when the author of *Airs, Waters, and Places* notes that in countries where people live on thin, ill-watered, and bare soils, and are adapted to seasonal changes, inhabitants are likely to be hard and well braced, of a blond rather than a dark complexion, and haughty and self-willed in their disposition and passions.[21]

The author of *Airs, Waters, and Places* offers empirical descriptions of the environment and patients and speculations about the potential links between them. The causal thinking appears to be that of his personal experience, as a traveling physician, about the geography and customs of the people that consult them. He is clearly biased in favor of the Greeks. For example, he declared that "the Asiatic race is feeble,"[22] and tolerates despotic governments. The Asiatic neighbors of the Greeks were the Babylonians and the Egyptians. The author deemed them to be more unwarlike and of gentler disposition than the Europeans because their seasons were more uniform.[23] He believed that in Greece, men were independent and warlike because the seasons in Greece were variable.

The authors of the Hippocratic Collection connected elements, celestial bodies, cardinal directions, organs, climates, seasons, colors, tastes, body fluids, and human experiences such as laughter or the feeling of pain to explain a person's health complaint. The Hippocratic treatises did not consider that patients who presented with similar symptoms suffered from the same disease. They did not group patients into diagnostic categories, count them, and compute averages and proportions. They described each patient's global experience as unique.

Daniel's Challenge

The Book of Daniel was originally written in Hebrew and Aramaic about 2,500 years ago in the period when the ancient Jews had been exiled from Palestine to Babylon. They lived as guests and prisoners of the Babylonian court. The Book of Daniel includes a passage that describes Daniel challenging Nebuchadnezzar, Babylon's ruler, to compare the effects of the diet of the Israelites with the food Babylonians ate. The text says that the diet Daniel and his compatriots ate was superior to the diet of the Babylonians.

King Nebuchadnezzar conquered Jerusalem and took "certain of the children of Israel, and of the king's seed, and of the princes" (Daniel 1:3–7) back to Babylon. Among them was Daniel. The king planned to assimilate these selected Israelites to the Babylonian culture and language. The Bible says that he selected them to be "good looking young men with perfect bodies [. . .] well-informed, intelligent and fit for service in the royal court." The king assigned his captives a daily allowance of food and wine from the royal table. Daniel considered that food inappropriate for the Jews. He wanted only vegetables and water. The guard feared that under such a diet the prisoners would lose weight and get sick. This prompted a shrewd reaction from Daniel, who told the guard, "Submit us to this test for ten days. Give us only vegetables to eat and water to drink; then compare our looks with those of the young men who have lived on the food assigned by the king and be guided in your treatment of us by

what you see." The guard agreed. At the end of ten days Daniel and his
countryman "looked healthier and were better nourished than all the
young men who had consumed the food assigned them by the king."[24]

According to epidemiologist Abraham Lilienfeld, this document,
found in the Old Testament in the first chapter of the Book of Daniel, is
"the earliest recorded account of a comparative study."[25]

Clinical Notes

We are aware of few documents from the Middle Ages and the Renaissance that are suggestive of quantified health events or of quantitative
comparisons. In the tenth century, the Ottoman Empire developed a
network of large hospitals staffed with physicians that may have provided
excellent conditions for quantifying medical events and comparing
groups.[26] The scholar Muhammad ibn Zakariya al-Rāzī (854–925 CE)
became a hospital director in both Rayy (his hometown, now a suburb of
Tehran) and in Baghdad.

As reported and translated by Peter Pormann, an expert in classics
and Graeco-Arabic studies, al-Rāzī listed the main symptoms of "brain
fever," which included heaviness, continuous pain in the head and neck,
yawning, severe insomnia, and extreme exhaustion. This list evokes the
modern diagnosis of meningitis. Al-Rāzī then wrote:

> So, when you see these symptoms, resort to bloodletting. For I
> once saved one group [of patients(ǧamāʿa)] by [bloodletting],
> whilst I intentionally [did not bleed] another group (ǧamāʿa),
> so as to remove the doubt from my opinion through this.
> Consequently, all of these [latter] contracted brain fever.[27]

Two more examples of al-Rāzī's use of the term "group" (ǧamāʿa) exist.
Given that the use of a control group was extraordinary then, Pormann
wondered whether al-Rāzī pioneered a notion of patient groups.

The two medical notes that follow are more recent than the example
from al-Rāzī. There is a letter that the eminent Italian poet Petrarch
wrote to his fellow poet Giovanni Boccaccio in 1364 in which he proposed a set of experiments to objectively evaluate medical expertise.

Latinist and historian Iain Donaldson has provided a new translation and interpretation of Petrarch's 1353 letter:

> If one hundred or one thousand men, of the same age and character and [eating the] same diet, one and all affected by the same disease, one half of them ask the advice of Doctors of the kind that there are in our time, and the other [half] without any Doctors should follow natural instinct and their own discernment then I have no doubt that of the former [half] many shall die and of the latter [half] many shall escape.[28]

The letter was titled "attack against a doctor" and expresses Petrarch's skepticism about medicine in the fourteenth century. The experiment is reminiscent of the trial Daniel proposed to the guard in Babylon except that Petrarch clearly described a fair comparison: the men in both groups should have the same age, character, and diet. Moreover, Petrarch seems to express the comparative experiment's outcome in terms of frequency ("many" shall die in one group vs. "many" shall survive in the other). An alternative explanation is that Petrarch used the Aristotelian logic that was common then. "Many shall die" was sufficient to prove that the "doctor's advice" was inefficient, while "many shall survive" proved that "instinct" and "discernments" were more effective.

The last example is provided by the mid-sixteenth-century Spanish surgeon Bartolomé Hidalgo de Agüero (1531–1597), who began a campaign for a change in the treatment of wounds.[29] The historian Carlos Solís has reported how Hidalgo de Agüero described the outcomes of his "dry" method, which relied on prompt cleaning and closure of the wound: the mortality was 4.4% (20/456). The alternative was the traditional "wet" method, which let the wound develop a thick form of pus that was widely considered essential for a healthy outcome. The wet methods had been associated with a mortality greater than 50% in the past. Hidalgo concluded that the dry method was superior to the wet method. In this before-and-after comparison, the "before" mortality is not exactly quantified.[30] Hidalgo may qualify as a precursor of quantified comparisons in the sixteenth century. He was a skilled surgeon if we trust that a prayer used in the Sevillian underworld before a knife fight was "En Dios me encomiendo, y en manos de Agüero" [In God I trust, and in Agüero's hands].[31]

Public Health in Antiquity

There is no clear indication that civilizations in antiquity understood the connection between any exposure that was not an immediate poison and an outcome. Consider the large public latrines provided by the government in the Roman Empire (31 BCE–476 CE). The buildings had multiple seats surrounding tubs that provided the water to clean the users. The water was brought to distribution tanks in Roman cities by huge aqueducts. It passed through settling tanks to eliminate sedimentary debris and then through covered channels. These sophisticated interventions gave urban residents access to clean water and enabled cities to grow. But for archeologist Piers D. Mitchell, latrines contributed to the spread of parasites.[32] Romans speculated that parasites spontaneously burst out of putrefied matter when the parasites experienced heat. They did not perceive any reason for changing the communal water often. They also used the human feces collected from towns to fertilize crops growing in the fields; this also may have spread viable parasite eggs to food. Mitchell's conclusion is sobering:

> We see the widespread presence of whipworm (*Trichuris trichiura*), roundworm (*Ascaris lumbricoides*) and *Entamoeba histolytica* that causes dysentery. This would suggest that the public sanitation measures were insufficient to protect the population from parasites spread by fecal contamination. Ectoparasites such as fleas, head lice, body lice, pubic lice and bed bugs were also present, and delousing combs have been found. The evidence fails to demonstrate that the Roman culture of regular bathing in the public baths reduced the prevalence of these parasites.[33]

Similar uses of human feces may explain endemics of intestinal maladies such as diarrhea and dysentery in Tenochtitlan, the capital of the Aztecs, in the fifteenth century, a city known for its impeccable cleanliness and its floating gardens. The city was built on a lake that absorbed sewage and detritus and was also a source of drinking water.[34]

The Romans and the Aztecs did not seem to have the concept of reaching beyond individual cases of illness to identify modes of transmission. If they had, they could have conducted a study similar to the epidemiological study the nineteenth-century British physician John Snow conducted in London that showed that cholera was transmitted by contaminated water. Snow compared two sets of Londoners. The members of one group drank water from areas of the River Thames that were polluted by the cholera bacillus. That group had much higher mortality from cholera during the epidemic of 1854 than a second group whose members lived in the same neighborhoods as the first group but who bought their water from a company that drew its water from less contaminated rural areas and filtered it.[35]

Romans could have compared the impact of changing communal water with varying frequencies and used that knowledge to improve the health of the public. Early societies lacked germ theory and antibiotics, but even without such tools, the spread of respiratory or gastrointestinal diseases can be controlled once one understands how these diseases are transmitted. Masks, physical distancing, hand washing, and clean water could have been implemented efficiently in human societies of the past. However, between the time of the Romans and the time of John Snow, there was a shift in perspective from thinking in terms of individuals to thinking in terms of a population that enabled public health officials to intervene to control specific diseases such as the plague, smallpox, and cholera.

Chapter 2 described the profound changes that occurred in the seventeenth century. New observational sciences emerged and deaths began to be counted using a specific infrastructure and specific expertise. These changes were part of a social, political, scientific, and cultural transformation of Western societies that were essential for the flourishing of the shift in perspective to population thinking.

Further Reading

This book is not a history of public health. It is a book about the perspective switch from the individual to the population level that is needed to contemplate the world as public health professionals do. I am not aware of another article or book on the same topic.

Useful Companions

Many articles and books are useful companions to this book and provide the contextual history of public health across the centuries visited in this book's chapters. George Rosen's *A History of Public Health*, although it is now seventy years old, remains the most erudite volume on the topic (Baltimore, MD: Johns Hopkins University Press, 1958; expanded edition, 1993). It covers the whole of human history until the 1950s. It is a pleasant read and provides a solid foundation for learning more about public health. The introduction of the 1993 edition by Elizabeth Fee reviews more recent developments in our understanding of the history of public health. Her introduction cites a rich literature of public health topics that have been published between 1957 and 1993. Fee explains that George Rosen's book remains unrivaled because of the fragmentation of public health history that occurred in the following decades. Rosen's traditional framework of Western civilization, a history that begins with the Greeks and the Romans and ends with twentieth-century America, began to look ethnocentric, old-fashioned, and limited from a contemporary point of view. "Yet," Fee wrote, "despite the fact that this [Rosen's] framework is no longer persuasive, we do not have a clear alternative." (*A History of Public Health* [1993], xxxix).

Rosen covered almost 4,000 years of public health, mostly in the Western world. In contrast, Henry E. Sigerist (1891–1957), director of Johns Hopkins University's Institute of the History of Medicine from 1932 until 1947, only covered antiquity in his *History of Medicine* (New York: Oxford University Press, 1951). He died before he could complete the rest of his outstanding work. His chapters on medicine in ancient Greece and Rome (vol. 1: *Primitive and Archaic Medicine*; vol. 2: *Early Greek, Indu and Persian Medicine*) are useful companions to the appendix to this volume.

To give public health practitioners access to the history of public health, George Rosen created a section of the *American Journal of Public Health* titled "Public Health Then and Now." Dozens of historians of public health have contributed to it over the last fifty years. Theodore Brown and I coedited an anthology of these articles for the 150th anniversary of the American Public Health Association titled *Public Health Then and Now: Landmark Papers from AJPH* (2022).

Virginia Berridge, Martin Gorsky and Alex Mold's textbook *Public Health in History* (Maidenhead: McGraw-Hill / Open University Press, 2011) gives a sense of what is a critical approach in history and the various ways primary and secondary documents can be interpreted. Their volume shows readers how to think about public health history.

Elizabeth Fee and Daniel M. Fox have co-edited two books about the AIDS epidemic: *AIDS: The Burdens of History* (Berkeley and Los Angeles: University of California Press, 1988) and *AIDS: The Making of a Chronic Disease* (Berkeley and Los Angeles: University of California Press, 1992). These volumes and their introductions are models of rigorous historiographical coverage of an acute public health crisis that was exacerbated by stigmatization and the blaming of victims. These books can inspire the historians of the COVID-19 pandemic.

Great histories have been written about the pandemics discussed in this book. For the bubonic plague, readers may wish to consult R. S. Gottfried's *The Black Death: Natural and Human Disaster in Medieval Europe* (New York: Free Press, 1983). Anthony Hopkins has written about smallpox in *The Greatest Killer: Smallpox in History* (Chicago: University of Chicago Press, 2002). Richard Evans's *Death in Hamburg: Society and Politics in the Cholera Years* (London: Penguin Books, 2005) is about the cholera pandemic that hit Hamburg in 1892 (described in chapter 4). John Barry's *The Great Influenza: The Epic Story of the Deadliest Plague in History* (New York: Penguin Books, 2005) is a history of the 1918 influenza pandemic. Marcus Grmek's *History of AIDS: Emergence and Origin of a Modern Pandemic* is well worth a reader's time (Princeton, NJ: Princeton University Press, 1990). Tricia Starks's *Cigarettes and Soviets: Smoking in the USSR* (Ithaca, NY: Cornell University Press, 2022) offers unique insights into both the history of tobacco and of public health in the USSR. An online source that is not a book but is rich and well done is the website "John Snow" that is hosted by the UCLA Department of Epidemiology (https://www.ph.ucla.edu/epi/snow.html).

Nancy Krieger has carved her place in the history of public health with her concept of ecoepidemiology. Her book *Epidemiology and the People's Health: Theory and Context* (New York: Oxford University Press, 2011) provides a solid scholarly history of how public health is practiced, and its connection with a broader political vision of justice.

For a general reference source about the different domains of public health, I strongly recommend the latest edition of *Maxcy-Rosenau-Last Public Health & Preventive Medicine* (New York: McGraw-Hill, 2022), an impressive compendium about the issues related to public health, including its subspecialities and the behavioral, biological, and social aspects of the field. I have a copy handily available on my shelf and consult it often, but it also exists electronically (https://accessmedicine.mhmedical.com/book.aspx?bookID=3078).

Finally, the American Public Health Association regularly publishes books on public health issues. The association's website (https://www

.apha.org/) provides a list of recent titles. Readings particularly relevant to contemporary social issues include *Gun Violence Prevention: A Public Health Approach*, edited by Linda Degutis and Howard Spivak (Washington DC: American Public Health Association, 2021) and *Racism: Science & Tools for the Public Health Professional*, by Chandra Ford, Derek Griffith, Marino Bruce, and Keon Gilbert (Washington, DC: APHA Press, 2019).

Notes

Prologue

1. Centers for Disease Control and Prevention, "Trends in Demographic Characteristics of People Receiving COVID-19 Vaccinations in the United States" and "Booster Vaccination Trends by Age, Sex, and Race/Ethnicity," accessed September 22, 2022, https://covid.cdc.gov/covid-data-tracker/#vaccinations_vacc-people-additional-dose-totalpop.

2. H. G. Rosenblum, J. Gee, R. Liu, P. L. Marquez, B. Zhang, P. Strid, et al., "Safety of mRNA Vaccines Administered during the Initial 6 Months of the US COVID-19 Vaccination Programme: An Observational Study of Reports to the Vaccine Adverse Event Reporting System and V-Safe," *The Lancet* 22(6) (2022): 802–812, https://doi.org/https://doi.org/10.1016/S1473-3099(22)00054-8.

3. According to the Centers for Disease Control and Prevention, only 5 people per million vaccinated in the United States experienced anaphylaxis after vaccination, 4 per million Americans who received Johnson & Johnson's Janssen vaccine experienced thrombosis with thrombocytopenia syndrome, and nine deaths were causally associated with Johnson & Johnson's Janssen COVID-19 vaccination. "Selected Adverse Effects Reported after COVID-19 Vaccination," https://www.cdc.gov/coronavirus/2019-ncov/vaccines/safety/adverse-events.html (as of 9/22/2022). Guillain-Barré syndrome was "a rare

side effect," accounting for 11 cases among the 483,000 who received Johnson & Johnson's Janssen vaccine and 36 cases among the 14,637,000 who received Pfizer-BioNTech's or Moderna's (mRNA) vaccines. Kayla E. Hanson, Kristin Goddard, Ned Lewis, et al., "Incidence of Guillain-Barré Syndrome after COVID-19 Vaccination in the Vaccine Safety Datalink," *JAMA Network Open* 5(4) (2022): e228879, https://doi.org/10.1001/jamanetworkopen.2022.8879. The CDC found "no increased risk of GBS after Pfizer-BioNTech or Moderna (mRNA COVID-19 vaccines)," https://www.cdc.gov /coronavirus/2019-ncov/vaccines/safety/adverse-events.html.

4. Texas Health and Human Services, "Texas Data Shows Unvaccinated People 20 Times More Likely to Die from COVID-19," news release, November 8, 2021, https://www.dshs.texas.gov/news/releases/2021 /20211108.aspx.

5. Worldwide, almost 20 million excess deaths were estimated to have been prevented in the first year after the introduction of vaccines. O. J. Watson, G. Barnsley, J. Toor, A. B. Hogan, P. Winskill, and A. C. Ghani, "Global Impact of the First Year of COVID-19 Vaccination: A Mathematical Modelling Study," *Lancet Infectious Diseases* 22(9) (2022): 1293–1302, https://doi.org/10.1016/S1473-3099(22)00320-6. In the United States, COVID-19 vaccination was estimated to prevent 27 million SARS-CoV-2 infections, 1.6 million COVID-19– associated hospitalizations, and 235,000 COVID-19–associated deaths among vaccinated persons 18 years or older from December 1, 2020, to September 30, 2021. M. K. Steele, A. Couture, C. Reed, et al., "Estimated Number of COVID-19 Infections, Hospitalizations, and Deaths Prevented among Vaccinated Persons in the US, December 2020 to September 2021," *JAMA Network Open* 5(8) (2022): e2220385, https://doi.org/10.1001/jamanetworkopen.2022.20385.

6. M.A. Rothstein and C. A. Hornung, "How Unrelated Health Events Can Hamper Covid Vaccination Efforts," *The Hill*, March 2, 2021, https://thehill.com/opinion/healthcare/541062-how-unrelated -health-events-can-hamper-covid-vaccination-efforts/.

7. M. Fauzia, "Fact Check: Not Likely That COVID-19 Vaccine Was Cause of Hank Aaron's Death," *USA Today*, January 26, 2021,

https://www.usatoday.com/story/news/factcheck/2021/01/26/fact
-check-hank-aaron-death-unlikely-result-covid-19-vaccine/6699
577002/.

8. M. Gladwell, *Outliers: The Story of Success* (New York: Little, Brown
    and Company, 2008), 10.

9. J. Graunt, *Natural and Political Observations Made upon the Bills
    of Mortality* [1662], ed. Walter J. Willcox (Baltimore, MD: Johns
    Hopkins Press, 1939).

10. V. Berridge, M. Gorsky, and A. Mold, *Public Health in History*
    (Maidenhead: McGraw-Hill/Open University Press, 2011),
    196.

11. Texas Health and Human Services, "Texas Data Shows Unvaccinated
    People 20 Times More Likely to Die from COVID-19," news release,
    November 8, 2021, https://www.dshs.texas.gov/news/releases/2021
    /20211108.aspx.

12. Graunt, *Natural and Political Observations*, II:15, 18.

13. G. Rose, "Sick Individuals and Sick Populations," *Int J Epidemiol*
    14(1) (2001): 32–38, https://doi.org/10.1093/ije/30.3.427.

14. G. Rose, *The Strategy of Preventive Medicine* (New York: Oxford
    University Press, 1993).

Chapter 1. Public Health

1. Centers for Disease Control and Prevention, "Public Opinion about
    Public Health—California and the United States, 1996. *MMWR
    Morb Mortal Wkly Rep* 47(4) (1998): 69–73; B. S. Levy, Creating the
    Future of Public Health: Values, Vision, and Leadership. *Am J Public
    Health* 88(2) (1998): 188–192.

2. Robert Wood Johnson Foundation and Harvard T. H. Chan School
    of Public Health, *The Public's Perspective on the United States Public
    Health Service*, May 20, 2021, https://cdn1.sph.harvard.edu/wp
    -content/uploads/sites/94/2021/05/RWJF-Harvard-Report_FINAL
    -051321.pdf.

3. A. Morabia, "What Is Public Health? An Interview with Former
    Governor John Kasich," *Am J Public Health* 112(4) (2022): 609–612,
    https://doi.org/10.2105/AJPH.2022.306751.

4. A. V. Roux, "On the Distinction—or Lack of Distinction—Between Population Health and Public Health," *Am J Public Health* 106(4) (2016): 619–620, https://doi.org/10.2105/AJPH.2016.303097.
5. M. A. Rothstein, "Rethinking the Meaning of Public Health," *J Law Med Ethics* 30(2) (2002): 144–149, https://doi.org/10.1111/j.1748 -720x.2002.tb00381.x.
6. As noted by historian Carlo Cipolla, "the concept of health organization as developed in the Renaissance Italian states eventually found systematic expression and elaboration in the late 1770s in the *System einer vollständigen Medizinischen Polizey* by Johann Peter Frank (1745–1821)." C. M. Cipolla, *Public Health and the Medical Profession in the Renaissance* (New York: Cambridge University Press. 1976), 65.
7. *System einer vollständigen medizinischen Polizey*, 9 vols. (Berlin, 1779–1827). The noun "Polizey" has sometimes been erroneously translated as "police." See also J. P. Frank, ed. and trans. H. E. Sigerist, "The People's Misery: Mother of Diseases (1790)," *Bull. Hist Med* 9(1) (1941): 81–100.
8. For a news report in English, see I. Foulkes, "Covid: Swiss Back Government on Covid Pass as Cases Surge," *BBC News*, November 28, 2021, https://www.bbc.com/news/world-europe-59380745.
9. Cipolla, *Public Health*, 66.
10. See M. Baker and D. Ivory, "Why Public Health Faces a Crisis across the U. S.," *New York Times*, October 18, 2021, https://www.nytimes .com/2021/10/18/us/coronavirus-public-health.html.

Chapter 2. Plague

1. G. Rosen, *A History of Public Health* (Baltimore, MD: Johns Hopkins University Press, 1958; expanded ed., 1993); D. Porter, *Health, Civilization, and the State: A History of Public Health from Ancient to Modern Times* (London: Routledge, 1999).
2. In *A Journal of the Plague Year*, the novelist Daniel Defoe described the progression of the disease: "Some were immediately overwhelmed with it, and it came to violent fevers, vomitings, insufferable headaches, pains in the back, and so up to ravings and ragings with those pains; others with swellings and tumors in the neck or

groin, or armpits, which till they could be broke put them into insufferable agonies and torment; while others, as I have observed, were silently infected, the fever preying upon their spirits insensibly, and they seeing little of it till they fell into swooning, and faintings, and death without pain." D. Defoe, *A Journal of the Plague Year* (New York: Penguin, 1960), 196.

3. "The Venetian authorities believed that if plague developed it would produce a general corruption of the air, and they promptly turned the infected away. Neither Venice nor Ragusa made any provisions for the isolation of the ill or the healthy who had contact with the disease. None of the original quarantine regulations set up at these ports were motivated by an idea of the specific contagiousness of the disease." Porter, *Health, Civilization, and the State,* 35.

4. K. L. Newman, "Shutt up: Bubonic Plague and Quarantine in Early Modern England," *J Soc Hist* 45(3) (2012): 809–834 (813–816), https://doi.org/10.1093/jsh/shr114.

5. S. J. Greenberg, "The 'Dreadful Visitation': Public Health and Public Awareness in Seventeenth-Century London," *Bull Med Libr Assoc* (4) (1997): 391–401.

6. K. Heitman, "Authority, Autonomy and the First London Bills of Mortality," *Centaurus* 62(2) (2020): 275–284 (281), https://doi.org/10.1111/1600-0498.12305.

7. Heitman, "Authority, Autonomy," 281.

8. C. H. Hull, introduction to *The Economic Writings of Sir William Petty,* ed. C. H. Hull (Cambridge: Cambridge University Press: 1899), lxxx–xci.

9. Bacon served as a Member of Parliament, the attorney general, the Lord Keeper of the Great Seal, and the Lord Chancellor before leaving politics in 1621. Over the next five years, he wrote twelve books and numerous essays and letters. M. B. Hesse, "Francis Bacon's Philosophy of Science," in *A Critical History of Western Philosophy,* ed. D. J. O'Connor (New York: Free Press, 1964), 141–152; J. Klein, "Francis Bacon," in *The Stanford Encyclopedia of Philosophy,* ed. E. N. Zalta (2012), http://plato.stanford.edu/archives/win2012/entries/francis-bacon.

10. Francis Bacon, *Works,* ed. J. Spedding, R. L. Ellis, and D. D. Heath, 3 vols. (1887), 3:394–395, cited in Klein, *Francis Bacon,* 12.

11. F. Bacon, *Accounts of Life and Death* (London, 1623), http://www.sirbacon.org/historylifedeath.htm. I would translate the Latin "Historia" by Accounts" and not, as usually seen, by "History".

12. The original (*Historia vitae et mortis* [London, 1623], 19-20) reads "8. De longevitate et brevitate vitae in hominibus, secundum victum, dietas, regimen vitae, exercitio, et similia, inquirito. Nam quatenus ad aerem, in quo vivunt et morantur homines, de eo in articulo superiore de locis habitationis inquiri debere intelligimus."

13. Eleanor J. Murray and her coauthors analyzed a seventeenth-century painting showing a relatively young man with long, unpowdered hair that could be a portrait of John Graunt. Historian Kristin Heitman found the painting. E. J. Murray, L. V. Farland, E. C. Caniglia, K. S. Dorans, N. C. DuPre, K. C. Hughes, I. Y. Kim, C. H. Pernar, L. J. Tanz, and R. M. Zack et al., "Is This a Portrait of John Graunt? An Art History Mystery," *Am J Epidemiol* 189(10) (2020): 1204–1207, https://doi.org/10.1093/aje/kwz212.

14. H. Westergaard, "Political Arithmetic in the Seventeenth Century," in H. Westergaard, ed., *Contributions to the History of Statistics* (New York: Kelley, 1969): 16–37.

15. P. Kreager, "New Light on Graunt," *Popul. Stud.* 1988. 42(1) (1988): 129–140, https://doi.org/ 10.1080/0032472031000143156.

16. Bills of mortality had one significant limitation: they recorded rites of passage for members of the Church of England; the births and deaths of people who did not follow Anglican rites were not included.

17. J. Graunt, *Natural and Political Observations Made upon the Bills of Mortality* (1662), ed. W. J. Willcox (Baltimore, MD: Johns Hopkins University Press, 1939), IV:12.

18. Graunt, *Natural and Political Observations,* II:19.

19. Graunt, *Natural and Political Observations,* II:15, 18.

20. "I conclude, that a clear knowledge of all these particulars, and many more, whereat I have shot but at rovers, is necessary in order to good, certain, and easie Government, and even to balance Parties and factions, both in Church and State. But whether the knowledge

thereof be necessary to many, or fit for others, than the Sovereign, and his chief Ministers, I leave to consideration." Graunt, *Natural and Political Observations*, Conclusion: 79.

21. Graunt, *Natural and Political Observations*, II:17.

22. M. Pfeffer, "Before Epidemiologists Began Modelling Disease, It Was the Job of Astrologers," *The Conversation*, May 19, 2020, https:// theconversation.com/before-epidemiologists-began-modelling -disease-it-was-the-job-of-astrologers-137895.

23. D. Bellhouse, "London Plague Statistics in 1665," *J. Official Statistics* 14(2) (1998): 207–234.

24. D. V. Glass, "John Graunt and His Natural and Political Observa- tions," *Proc R Soc Lond B Biol Sci* 159(974) (1963): 1–37, http://www .jstor.org/stable/90480.

25. P. Slack, "The Disappearance of Plague: An Alternative View," *Econ Hist Rev* 34(3) (1981): 469–476, https://doi.org/10.2307/2595884.

26. J. N. Biraben, *Les hommes et la peste en France et dans les pays européens et méditerranéens* (Paris: Mouton, 1975); A. B. Appleby, "The Disappearance of Plague: A Continuing Puzzle," *Econ Hist Rev* 1980. 33 (1980): 161–173, https://doi.org/10.1111/j.1468-0289.1980. tb01821.x.

27. K. Pearson, *The History of Statistics in the 17th and 18th Centuries against the Changing Background of Intellectual, Scientific and Religious Thought*, ed. E. S. Pearson (London: Charles Griffin, 1978); M. Greenwood, "Medical Statistics from Graunt to Farr," *Biometrika* 32(2) (1941): 101–127, https://doi.org/10.2307/2332126.

28. Graunt, *Natural and Political Observations*, Conclusion: 3.

Chapter 3. Smallpox

1. W. A. Guy, "Two Hundred and Fifty Years of Small Pox in London," *J Stat Soc of London* 45(3) (1882): 399–443, https://doi.org /10.2307/2979319; C. Creighton, *A History of Epidemics in Britain*, 2: *From the Extinction of Plague to the Present Time* (London: Cambridge University Press, 1894); J. Koopman, "Epidemiology. Controlling Smallpox" *Science* 298(5597) (2002): 1342–1344, https://doi.org/10.1126/science.1079370.

2. Centers for Disease Control and Prevention, "How Does Smallpox Spread?" last reviewed June 7, 2016, https://www.cdc.gov/smallpox /transmission/index.html.

3. W. H. McNeill, *Plagues and Peoples* (New York: Anchor Books, 1977), 55, 119.

4. D. R. Hopkins, *The Greatest Killer: Smallpox in History* (Chicago: University of Chicago Press, 2002), 14.

5. C. C. Mann, *1491: New Revelations of the Americas before Columbus* (New York: Vintage Books, 2006).

6. J. Duffy, "Smallpox and the Indians in the American Colonies," *Bull Hist Med* 25(4) (1951): 324–341, https://www.jstor.org/stable /44443622.

7. K. Dewhurst, "Sydenham's Original Treatise on Smallpox with a Preface, and Dedication to the Earl of Shaftesbury, by John Locke," *Med Hist* 3(4) (1959): 278–302 (290), https://doi.org/doi: 10.1017 /s0025727300024790.

8. A. W. Boylston, *Defying Providence: Smallpox and the Forgotten 18th Century Medical Revolution* (North Charleston, SC: Great-space, 2012), 12

9. Boylston, *Defying Providence*, 12–13.

10. A. Boylston, "The Origins of Inoculation," *J R Soc Med.* 105(7) (2012): 309–313, https://doi.org/10.1258/jrsm.2012.12k044.

11. "The small-pox, so fatal, and so general amongst us, is here entirely harmless, by the invention of engrafting, which is the term they give it. There is a set of old women, who make it their business to perform the operation, every autumn, in the month of September, when the great heat is abated. People send to one another to know if any of their family has a mind to have the small-pox; they make parties for this purpose, and when they are met (commonly fifteen or sixteen together) the old woman comes with a nut-shell full of the matter of the best sort of small-pox, and asks what vein you please to have opened. She immediately rips open that you offer to her, with a large needle (which gives you no more pain than a common scratch) and puts into the vein as much matter as can lie upon the head of her needle, and after that, binds up the little wound with a hollow bit

of shell, and in this manner opens four or five veins. [. . .] The children or young patients play together all the rest of the day, and are in perfect health to the eighth. Then the fever begins to seize them, and they keep their beds two days, very seldom three. They have very rarely above twenty or thirty [spots] in their faces, which never mark, and in eight days time they are as well as before their illness. Where they are wounded, there remains running sores during the distemper, which I don't doubt is a great relief to it. [. . .] There is no example of any one that has died in it, and you may believe I am well satisfied of the safety of this experiment, since I intend to try it on my dear little son." Lady Montagu to Mrs. S. C., 1717, letter 36 in *Lady Mary Wortley Montagu, Letters of the Right Honourable Lady M—y W—y M—e: Written during Her Travels in Europe, Asia and Africa*, vol. 1 (Aix: Anthony Henricy, 1796), 167–169.

12. Boylston, *Defying Providence*, 23.

13. A. M. Kass, "Boston's Historic Smallpox Epidemic," *Mass Hist Rev* 14(1) (2012): 1–51 (30), https://doi.org/10.5224/masshistrevi.14.1 .0001.

14. L. Farmer, "The Smallpox Inoculation Controversy and the Boston Press, 1721-2," *Bull N Y Acad Med* 34(9) (1958): 599–608.

15. Kass, "Boston's Historic Smallpox Epidemic," 30.

16. Mather, quoted in Robert Tindol, "Getting the Pox off All Their Houses: Cotton Mather and the Rhetoric of Puritan Science," *Early American Lit* 46, no. 1 (2011): 1–23 (8), https://doi.org/10.1353 /eal.2011.0002.

17. Kass, "Boston's Historic Smallpox Epidemic," 20.

18. S. Buhr, "To Inoculate or Not to Inoculate? The Debate and the Smallpox Epidemic of Boston in 1721," *Constructing the Past* 1(1) (2000): 61–67 (63).

19. T. M. Brown, "Medicine in the Shadow of the *Principia*," *J Hist Ideas* 48(4) (1987): 629–648, https://doi.org/10.2307/2709691.

20. J. Jurin, *An Account of the Success of Inoculating the Small Pox in Great Britain: With a Comparison between the Miscarriages in that Practice, and the Mortality of the Natural Small-Pox* (London: Peele, 1724), 3, http://name.umdl.umich.edu/004794581.0001.000.

21. "For the past ten years, there have died of the smallpox, within the bills of mortality, in average 2,287 persons per year. Let us now consider what may be the consequence, in case inoculation should hereafter become a general practice. If we allow all the opposers of inoculation contend for, we shall find one in 49 to die of inoculation, and in the natural way, we have shown it to be one in six: it follows, that if we substitute inoculation for the natural way, the number of the dead would be reduced seven parts in eight, and consequently 2,000 persons, that are yearly cut off, within the bills of mortality alone, and those generally in the beginning, or prime of life, might be preserved to their King and country. Let the warm opposers of inoculation, lay their hands upon their hearts, and consider, whether the saving of so many lives, be contrary to any precept of law, or gospel. We have been told indeed, and from the pulpit too, that this practice came from the devil: but if it prove thus beneficial and salutary to mankind, I, for my part, shall make no scruple of ascribing it to a greater and a better author; and undoubtedly, all sober and thinking persons will judge and believe, that the making known to the world, a method of preserving their lives from one of the most terrible diseases in nature, can be owing to no other, than the kind and tender providence of the great creator and preserver of mankind." Jurin, *An Account of the Success of Inoculating the Small Pox*, 32–33.

22. Jurin, *An Account of the Success of Inoculating the Small Pox*, 7.

23. Jurin, Advertisement, in *An Account of the Success of Inoculating the Small Pox*, [unnumbered page].

24. The data come from several reports listed in Jurin, *An Account of the Success of Inoculating the Small Pox*, 7.

25. Jurin, *An Account of the Success of Inoculating the Small Pox*, 32.

26. Boylston, *Defying Providence*, 145.

27. B. Franklin, "Preface to Dr. Heberden's Pamphlet on Inoculation," February 16, 1759, in *The Papers of Benjamin Franklin*, 8: *April 1, 1758, through December 31, 1759*, ed. Leonard W. Labaree (New Haven, CT: Yale University Press, 1965), 281–286, https://founders.archives.gov/documents/Franklin/01-08-02-0073.

28. *The Autobiography of Benjamin Franklin & Selections from His Other Writings* (New York: Modern Library, 1950), 113–114.

29. Franklin, "Preface to Dr. Heberden's Pamphlet on Inoculation."

30. Franklin, "Preface to Dr. Heberden's Pamphlet on Inoculation."

31. During a smallpox epidemic, doctors "probably could not so particularly attend to the circumstances of the patients offered for Inoculation," Franklin wrote. "Preface to Dr. Heberden's Pamphlet on Inoculation."

32. H. Markel, "Life, Liberty and the Pursuit of Vaccines," *New York Times*, March 11, 2001, https://www.nytimes.com/2011/03/01/health/01smallpox.html.

33. Frequently cited sources are chapter 10 of James E. Gibson, *Dr. Bodo Otto and the Medical Background of the American Revolution* (Baltimore: Charles C. Thomas, 1937); and H. Thursfield, "Smallpox in the American War of Independence," *Ann Med Hist* 2(4) (1940): 312–318, https://www.ncbi.nlm.nih.gov/pmc/articles/PMC7942582/pdf/annmedhist148632-0054.pdf. These two documents don't cite their sources and are used as original sources by many authors, including Donald Hopkins (*The Greatest Killer: Smallpox in History* [Chicago: University of Chicago Press, 2002]) and Arthur Boylston (*Defying Providence*). The inoculation of the Continental Army was a complex and hesitating process that probably took a couple of years, as per the better-documented A. M. Becker, "Smallpox in Washington's Army: Strategic Implications of the Disease during the American Revolutionary War," *J Military History* 68(2) (2004): 381–430, http://www.jstor.org/stable/3397473.

34. Gibson, *Dr. Bodo Otto*, 99.

35. John Adams to Abigail Adams, June 26, 1776, cited by Becker, "Smallpox in Washington's Army," 420.

36. In February 1777 George Washington wrote: "The deplorable and melancholy situation, to which one of our Armies was reduced last Campaign by the small Pox . . . has determined me . . . to introduce inoculation immediately." George Washington to Nicholas Cooke, February 10, 1777, in Fitzpatrick, *Writings of George Washington*, 7:131 cited by Becker, "Smallpox in Washington's Army," 422.

37. Boylston, *Defying Providence*, 212.
38. Rosen, *A History of Public Health* (1993), 164.
39. A. Rusnock, "Catching Cowpox: The Early Spread of Smallpox Vaccination, 1798–1810," *Bull Hist Med* 83(1) (2009): 17–36, https://doi.org/10.1353/bhm.0.0160.
40. A. W. Boylston, "The Origins of Vaccination: No Inoculation, No Vaccination," *J R Soc Med* 106(10) (2013) :395–398, https://doi.org/10.1177/0141076813499293.
41. E. Jenner, *An Inquiry Into the Causes and Effects of the Variolae Vaccinae: A Disease Discovered in Some of the Western Counties of England, Particularly Gloucestershire, and Known by the Name of the Cow Pox* (London: Sampson Low, 1798), 45
42. Boylston, *Defying Providence*, chap. 17.
43. D. Tarantola, "DA Henderson, Smallpox Eradicator," *Am J Public Health* 106(11) (2016): 1895, https://doi.org/10.2105/AJPH.2016.303477.
44. D. R. Hopkins, "Smallpox: Ten Years Gone," *Am J Public Health* 78(12) (1988): 1589–1595, https://doi.org/10.2105/ajph.78.12.1589.

Chapter 4. Cholera

1. R. J. Evans, "Epidemics and Revolutions: Cholera in Nineteenth-Century Europe," *Past & Present* 120 (1988): 123–146, https://doi.org/10.1093/past/120.1.123
2. E. Hobsbawm, *The Age of Revolution: 1789–1848* (New York: Vintage Books, 1996).
3. M. Benoiston de Chateauneuf, Commission instituée pour recueillir les faits relatifs à l'invasion et aux effets du choléra-morbus dans le département de la Seine, Préfecture de police, Seine. *Rapport sur la marche et les effets du choléra-morbus dans Paris et les communes rurales du département de la Seine: année 1832* (Paris: Imprimerie Royale, 1834), https://gallica.bnf.fr/ark:/12148/bpt6k842918.image.
4. A. F. La Berge, "Edwin Chadwick and the French Connection," *Bull Hist Med.* 62, no. 1 (1988): 27, https://www.jstor.org/stable/44449291.
5. All the data and dates in this paragraph are in chapter 3 of the report.

6. *Rapport sur la marche et les effets du choléra-morbus,* 41–42.

7. *Rapport sur la marche et les effets du choléra-morbus,* 45.

8. *Rapport sur la marche et les effets du choléra-morbus,* 48–49.

9. C. Rollet and A. Souriac, "Épidémies et mentalités: Le choléra de 1832 en Seine-et-Oise," *Annales. Économies, Sociétés, Civilisations* 29(4) (1974): 935–965, https://www.jstor.org/stable/27579354.

10. G. Rosen, *A History of Public Health,* expanded ed. (Baltimore, MD: Johns Hopkins University Press, 1993), chap. 6.

11. R. J. Davenport, "Urbanization and Mortality in Britain, c. 1800–50," *Econ Hist Rev* 73(2) (2020): 455–485, https://doi.org/10.1111/ehr.12964.

12. See the essays prefaced and translated by Henry E. Sigerist in M. von Pettenkofer, *The Value of Health to a City: Two Lectures Delivered in 1873 by Max von Pettenkofer* (Baltimore, MD: Johns Hopkins University Press, 1941).

13. R. Gehrmann, "Infant Mortality in Germany in the 19th Century," *Comparative Population Studies* 36(4) (2011): 839–868, https://doi.org/10.12765/CPoS-2011-22.

14. A. Morabia, *Enigmas of Health and Disease: How Epidemiology Helps Unravel Scientific Mysteries* (New York: Columbia University Press, 2014), 21–29.

15. [Report of the London] "Epidemiological Society," November 7, 1864, *British Medical Journal* 2, no. 203 (1864): 587.

16. R. J. Evans, "Epidemics and Revolutions: Cholera in Nineteenth-Century Europe," *Past & Present* (120) (1988): 123–146 (125), https://www.jstor.org/stable/650924.

17. W. Farr, "Influence of Elevation on the Fatality of Cholera," *J Stat Soc London* 15(2) (1852): 155–183, https://www.jstor.org/stable/pdf/2338305.pdf.

18. J. Snow, *Snow on Cholera* (New York: The Commonwealth Fund, 1936), 97–98.

19. N. Paneth, P. Vinten-Johansen, H. Brody, and M. Rip, "A Rivalry of Foulness: Official and Unofficial Investigations of the London Cholera Epidemic of 1854," *Am J Public Health* 88(10) (1998): 1545–1553, https://doi.org/10.2105/ajph.88.10.1545.

20. Paneth et al., "A Rivalry of Foulness."

21. J. Snow, *On the Mode of Communication of Cholera*. 2nd ed. (London: Churchill, 1855).

22. Snow, *On the Mode of Communication of Cholera*.

23. J. P. Vandenbroucke, H. M. Eelkman Rooda, and H. Beukers, "Who Made John Snow a Hero?" *Am J Epidemiol* 133(10) (1991): 967–973, https://doi.org/10.1093/oxfordjournals.aje.a115816.

24. R. J. Evans, *Death in Hamburg: Society and Politics in the Cholera Years* (London: Penguin Books, 2005), 294–295

25. Evans, *Death in Hamburg*, 293.

26. The belief in miasmas did not disappear overnight, but it became irreversible after the Hamburg debacle. As early as 1893, Pettenkofer was described as "completely isolated" in the medical profession. Evans, *Death in Hamburg*, 503.

27. Evans, *Death in Hamburg*, 564

28. Rosen, *A History of Public Health* (1993), 202.

29. C. Hamlin, *Public Health and Social Justice in the Age of Chadwick* (Cambridge: Cambridge University Press, 1997); C. Hamlin, "'Cholera Forcing': The Myth of the Good Epidemic and the Coming of Good Water," *Am J Public Health* 99(11) (2009): 1946–1954, https//doi.org/10.2105/AJPH.2009.165688.

30. "A clue to an understanding of the ascendancy of anticontagionism during this period is provided by the observation that it coincides with the rise of liberalism. Anticontagionists in many instances were liberal reformers who fought for individual freedom against despotism and reaction." Rosen, *A History of Public Health* (1993), 265–266.

31. A. L. Fairchild, David Rosner, James Colgrove, Ronald Bayer, and L. P. Fried et al., "The EXODUS of Public Health. What History Can Tell Us about the Future," *Am J Public Health* 100(1) (2010): 54–63 (56), https://doi.org/10.2105/AJPH.2009.163956.

32. See the memorial volume edited by Noel Humphreys for the Sanitary Insitute of Great Britain in 1885, reproduced in M. Susser and A. Adelstein, *Vital Statistics: A Memorial Volume of Selections from the Reports and Writings of William Farr* (Metuchen, NJ:

Scarecrow Press, 1975). See also the lectures by Max von Pettenkofer mentioned in note 11 of this chapter.

33. Rosen, *A History of Public Health* (1993), 191.

34. Fairchild et al., "The EXODUS of Public Health."

35. M. Susser and Z. Stein, *Eras in Epidemiology* (New York: Oxford University Press, 2009).

36. J. Lister, "Effects of the Antiseptic System of Treatment upon the Salubrity of a Surgical Hospital," *The Lancet* 95(2419) (1870) 40–42, https://doi.org/10.1016/S0140-6736(02)31303-5.

37. A. Hardy, *The Epidemic Streets: Infectious Disease and the Rise of Preventive Medicine. 1856-1900* (Oxford: Clarendon Press, 1993); A. Hardy, "Methods of Outbreak Investigation in the 'Era of Bacteriology,' 1880-1920," *Soz Präventivmed* 46(6) (2001): 355–360, https://doi.org/10.1007/BF01321661.

38. H. T. Bulstrode, *Dr. H. Timbrell Bulstrode's Report to the Local Government Board upon Alleged Oyster-Borne Enteric Fever and Other Illness following the Mayoral Banquets at Winchester and Southampton, and upon Enteric Fever Occurring Simultaneously Elsewhere, and Also Ascribed to Oysters* (London: Darling & Son, 1902); A. Morabia and A. Hardy, "The Pioneering Use of a Questionnaire to Investigate a Food Borne Disease Outbreak in Early 20th Century Britain," *J Epidemiol Community Health* 59(2) (2005): 94–99, https://doi.org/10.1136/jech.2004.025700.

39. A. Morabia, B. Rubenstein, and C. G. Victora, "Epidemiology and Public Health in 1906 England: Arthur Newsholme's Methodological Innovation to Study Breastfeeding and Fatal Diarrhea,"*Am J Public Health* 103(7) (2013): e17–e22; A. Newsholme, "Domestic Infection in Relation to Epidemic Diarrhoea," *J Hyg* (London) 6(2) (1906): 139–148, https://doi.org/10.1017/s0022172400002783.

Chapter 5. Tuberculosis

1. J. E. Abrams, "'Spitting Is Dangerous, Indecent, and against the Law!' Legislating Health Behavior during the American Tuberculosis Crusade," *J Hist Med Allied Sci* 68(3) (2013): 416–450, https://doi.org/ 10.1093/jhmas/jrr073.

2. T. F. Brewer, "Preventing Tuberculosis with Bacillus Calmette-Guérin Vaccine: A Meta-Analysis of the Literature," *Clin Infect Dis* 31(Suppl 3) (2000): S64–S67, https://doi.org/10.1086/314072.

3. M. S. Pernick, "Eugenics and Public Health in American History," *Am J Public Health* 87(11) (1997): 1767–1772, https://doi.org /10.2105/ajph.87.11.1767.

4. J. A. Tobey, review of H. H. Laughlin, *Historical, Legal, and Statistical Review of Eugenical Sterilization in the United States* (New Haven, American Eugenics Society, 1926), *Am J Public Health* 16(7) (1926): 725–726, https://ajph.aphapublications.org/doi/pdf/10.2105 /AJPH.16.7.725-b

5. A. M. Stern [University of Michigan, Institute for Healthcare Policy and Innovation], "Forced Sterilization Policies in the US Targeted Minorities and Those with Disabilities–And Lasted into the 21st Century," September 20, 2020, https://ihpi.umich.edu/news /forced-sterilization-policies-us-targeted-minorities-and-those -disabilities-and-lasted-21st.

6. A. M. Stern, "Making Better Babies: Public Health and Race Betterment in Indiana, 1920–1935," *Am J Public Health* 92(5) (2002): 742–752, https://doi.org/10.2105/ajph.92.5.742.

7. A. Morabia and R. Guthold, "Wilhelm Weinberg's 1913 Large Retrospective Cohort Study: A Rediscovery," *Am J Epidemiol* 165 (7) (2007): 727–733, table 2, https://doi.org/10.1093/aje/kwk062.

8. P. Weindling, *Health, Race, and German Politics between National Unification and Nazism, 1870–1945* (New York: Cambridge University Press, 1989).

9. R. Rogaski, "The Manchurian Plague and COVID-19: China, the United States, and the 'Sick Man,' Then and Now. *Am J Public Health* 111(3) (2021): 423–429, https://doi.org/10.2105/AJPH .2020.305960.

10. "Streptomycin Treatment of Pulmonary Tuberculosis," *BMJ* 2(4582) (1948): 769–782, https://www.bmj.com/content/2/4582/769.

11. On the design of the trial and its impact on clinical medicine, see A. Yoshioka, "The Randomized Controlled Trial of Streptomycin," in *The Oxford Textbook of Clinical Research Ethics,* ed. E. J. Emanuel,

C. Grady, R. A. Crouch, R. K. Lie, F. G. Miller, and D. Wendler, 46–60 (Oxford: University Press Oxford, 2008).

12. World Health Organization, "Tuberculosis: Key Facts," October 14, 2021, https://www.who.int/news-room/fact-sheets/detail/tuberculosis.

13. The new US schools focused on biomedical research without considering the social and economic contexts for their work. They were not interested in social or economic reforms. Institute of Medicine, Committee on Educating Public Health Professionals for the 21st Century, *Who Will Keep the Public Healthy? Educating Public Health Professionals for the 21st Century*, ed. K. Gebbie, L. Rosenstock, and L. Hernandez (Washington, DC: National Academies Press, 2003).

14. For a history of epidemiology and medical statistics at the London School of Hygiene and Tropical Medicine, see chapter 4 in Lise Wilkinson and Anne Hardy, *Prevention and Cure: The London School of Hygiene & Tropical Medicine: A 20th Century Quest for Global Public Health* (London: Kegan Paul, 2001), 92–124.

Chapter 6. Cancer and Cardiovascular Diseases

1. A. Morabia, "Why Does Influenza Hit the Poor More than the Rich? A 1931 Social Epidemiology Article That Broke New Ground in the History of Confounding, Mediation, and Interaction," *Am J Epidemiol* 190(11) (2021): 2235–2241, https://doi.org/10.1093/aje/kwab198.

2. E. Sydenstricker, Statistics of Morbidity, *Milbank Q.* 10(2) (1932): 101–119, https://doi.org/10.2307/3347577; G. Weisz, "Epidemiology and Health Care Reform: The National Health Survey of 1935–1936," *Am J Public Health* 101(3) (2011): 438–447, https://doi.org/10.2105/AJPH.2010.196519.

3. See the following epidemiologic milestones: J. Lane-Claypon, *A Further Report on Cancer of the Breast, with Special Reference to Its Associated Antecedent Conditions*, Ministry of Health Reports on Public Health and Medical Subjects, no. 32 (London, HMSO, 1926), 1–189; F. L. Hoffman, "Cancer and Smoking Habits," *Ann. Surg.*

93(1) (1931): 50–67, https://doi.org/ 10.1097/00000658-193101 000-00009; J. P. English, F. A. Willius, and J. Berkson, "Tobacco and Coronary Disease," *J Am Med Assoc* 115(16) (1940): 1327–1328, https://doi.org/10.1001/jama.1940.02810420013004.

4. A wonderful book about the role of tobacco during wars is T. Starks, *Cigarettes and Soviets: Smoking in the USSR* (Ithaca, NY: Cornell University Press, 2022).

5. A. H. Roffo, "Durch Tabak beim Kaninchen entwickeltes Carcinom," *J Cancer Res Clin Oncol* 33(1) (1931): 321–332, https://doi.org /10.1007/BF01792286.

6. Hoffman, "Cancer and Smoking Habits."

7. "The most interesting effects of smoking are those which occur to the central nervous system. Like alcohol, tobacco is often called a 'stimulant'—it is said to pep you up—but instead, much like alcohol, it is mainly the opposite: a sedative. Professor Mendenhall points out that it has an effect similar to that of rest, and he called cigarettes 'a package of rest.' This is probably the main basis of the smoking habits although in many cases the 'feel' of the cigarette or pipe or cigar in the mouth is the basis of the same habit, on its own account. The source of the 'rest' in tobacco is the nicotine in it." A. G. Ingalls, "If You Smoke," *Sci Am* 154(6) (1936): 310–313, http://www .jstor.org/stable/26144809.

8. A. M. Brandt, *The Cigarette Century: The Rise, Fall and Deadly Persistence of the Product That Defined America* (New York: Basic Books, 2007); R. N. Proctor, *Golden Holocaust: Origins of the Cigarette Catastrophe and the Case for Abolition* (Berkeley: University of California Press, 2011).

9. H. F. Dorn, "The Relationship of Cancer of the Lung and the Use of Tobacco," *Am Statistician*, 8(5) (1954): 7–13, https://doi.org/10.1080 /00031305.1954.10482762.

10. R. Doll and A. B. Hill, "The Mortality of Doctors in Relation to Their Smoking Habits:A Preliminary Report," *Br Med J* 1(4877) (1954): 1451–1455, https://doi.org/10.1136/bmj.328.7455.1529.

11. E. C. Hammond and D. Horn, "The Relationship between Human Smoking Habits and Death Rates: A Follow-Up Study of 187,766

Men," *J Am Med Assoc* 155(15) (1954): 1316–1328, https://doi.org
/10.1001/jama.1954.03690330020006.

12. M. N. Gardner and A.M. Brandt, "'The Doctors' Choice Is America's
Choice': The Physician in US Cigarette Advertisements, 1930–1953,"
Am J Public Health 96(2) (2006): 222–232. https://doi.org/10.2105
/AJPH.2005.066654.

13. J. Cornfield, "Recent Methodological Contributions to Clinical
Trials,"*Am J Epidemiol* 104(4) (1976): 408–421 (408), https://doi
.org/10.1093/oxfordjournals.aje.a112313.

14. R. A. Fisher, *The Design of Experiments* (Edinburgh: Oliver and
Boyd, 1935).

15. Fisher, *The Design of Experiments,* 11.

16. A. Morabia, "Has Epidemiology Become Infatuated with Methods?
A Historical Perspective on the Place of Methods during the
Classical (1945–1965) Phase of Epidemiology," *Ann Rev Public
Health* 36 (2015): 69–88, https://doi.org/10.1146/annurev
-publhealth-031914-122403.

17. Royal College of Physicians of London, *Smoking and Health:
Summary Report of the Royal College of Physicians of London on
Smoking in Relation to Cancer of the Lung and Other Diseases*
(London: Pitman, 1962).

18. Royal College of Physicians of London, *Smoking and Health,* 27.

19. R. Pearl, "Tobacco Smoking and Longevity," *Science* 87(2254) (1938):
216–217, https://doi.org/10.1126/science.87.2253.216; R. Doll and
A. B. Hill, "Mortality in Relation to Smoking: Ten Years' Observations of British Doctors," *Br Med J* 1(5396) (1964): 1399–1410,
1460–1467, https://doi.org/10.1136/bmj.1.5395.1399.

20. O. W. Brawley, T. J. Glynn, F. R. Khuri, R. C. Wender, and J. R.
Seffrin, "The First Surgeon General's Report on Smoking and
Health: The 50th Anniversary," *CA: A Cancer Journal for Clinicians*
64(1) (2014), https://doi.org/10.3322/caac.21210.

21. President John F. Kennedy, Press Conference 34 (May 23, 1962),
https://www.youtube.com/watch?v=dT6ACaxRuLQ (audio).

22. Brawley et al., "The First Surgeon General's Report on Smoking and
Health."

23. United States Surgeon General's Advisory Committee on Smoking and Health, *Smoking and Health* (Washington, DC: Government Printing Office, 1964).

24. R. Kluger, *Ashes to Ashes: America's Hundred-Year Cigarette War, the Public Health, and the Unabashed Triumph of Philip Morris* (New York: Vintage, 1997), 242–244.

25. United States Surgeon General's Advisory Committee on Smoking and Health, *Smoking and Health*, 185.

26. United States Surgeon General's Advisory Committee on Smoking and Health, *Smoking and Health*, 175–76, 185

27. Kluger, *Ashes to Ashes*, 252.

28. K. E. Warner, "50 Years since the First Surgeon General's Report on Smoking and Health: A Happy Anniversary?" *Am J Public Health* 104(1) (2014): 5–8, https://doi.org/10.2105/AJPH.2013.301722

29. Morabia, "Has Epidemiology Become Infatuated with Methods?"

30. "Flight Attendants, Big Tobacco Settle Secondhand-Smoke Case," *Wall Street Journal*, October 10, 1997, https://www.wsj.com/articles/SB876496061432501000.

31. Americans for Nonsmokers' Rights Foundation, "Overview List: How Many Smokefree and Other Tobacco-Related Laws?" (January 1, 2023), www.no-smoke.org/pdf/mediaordlist.pdf, accessed February 2, 2023.

32. A. B. Hill, "The Environment and Disease: Association or Causation?" *Proc Royal Soc Med* 58(5) (1965): 295–300, https://www.ncbi.nlm.nih.gov/pmc/articles/PMC2626428/.

33. A. Morabia, "Hume, Mill, Hill, and the Sui Generis Epidemiologic Approach to Causal Inference," *Am J Epidemiol* 178(10) (2013): 1526–1532, https://doi.org/10.1093/aje/kwt223.

34. R. A. Fisher, *Smoking, The Cancer Controversy: Some Attempts to Assess the Evidence* (Edinburgh: Oliver and Boyd, 1959).

35. R.A. Fisher, "Cigarettes, Cancer, and Statistics," *Centennial Review of Arts and Sciences* 2 (1958): 164, http://www.jstor.org/stable/23737529.

36. Fisher, *Smoking, The Cancer Controversy*, 39.

37. Doll and Hill, "The Mortality of Doctors in Relation to Their Smoking Habits, 1461.

38. W. Rothstein, *Public Health and the Risk Factor: A History of an Uneven Medical Revolution* (Rochester, NY: University of Rochester Press, 2003).

39. W. B. Kannel, T. R. Dawber, A. Kagan, N. Revotskie, and J. Stokes 3rd, "Factors of Risk in the Development of Coronary Heart Disease—Six Year Follow-Up Experience: The Framingham Study," *Ann Intern Med* 55 (1961): 33–50, https://doi.org/10.7326/0003 -4819-55-1-33; T. R. Dawber, *The Framingham Study: The Epidemiology of Atherosclerotic Disease* (Cambridge, MA: Harvard University Press, 1980); G. M. Oppenheimer, "Becoming the Framingham Study, 1947–1950," *Am J Public Health* 95(4) (2005): 602–610, https://doi.org/10.2105/AJPH.2003.026419.

40. T. R. Dawber, F. E. Moore, and G. V. Mann, "Coronary Heart Disease in the Framingham Study," *Am J Public Health Nations Health* 47(4/2) (1957): 4–24, https://doi.org/10.2105/ajph.47.4_pt_2.4.

41. D. M. Fox, *Power and Illness: The Failure and Future of American Health Policy* (Berkeley: University of California Press, 1993).

42. T. R. Dawber, G. F. Meadors, and F. E. Moore Jr., "Epidemiological Approaches to Heart Disease: The Framingham Study," *Am J Public Health* 41(3) (1951): 279–281 (280), 10.2105/ajph.41.3.279.

43. Dawber, Moore, and Mann, "Coronary Heart Disease in the Framingham Study."

44. Dawber, Moore, and Mann, "Coronary Heart Disease in the Framingham Study," 18, table 13:

BLOOD PRESSURE	CHOLESTEROL	HEART DISEASE (NO.)	POPULATION (NO.)	4-YEAR RISK (%)
Norm	Norm	1	98	0.01
Norm	High	9	112	0.08
High	Norm	3	47	0.06
High	High	5	17	0.29

45. A. Keys, "Coronary Heart Disease in Seven Countries," *Nutrition* 13(3) (1970): 250–252, https://doi.org/10.1016/s0899-9007(96) 00410-8.

46. When Henry Blackburn was asked about why women were not included in the study, he responded that an exponentially larger study would not have been possible at the time: "If the Seven Countries Study preplanning found that cohort sizes of 600 to 800 middle-aged men would be required to produce enough CVD events to compare, rationally, differences in 10-year cardiovascular disease rates for men, longitudinal studies would have to include 4–5 times larger population samples to get such evidence for women" (personal communication, March 28, 2022).

47. University of Minnesota, "Heart Attack Prevention: A History of Cardiovascular Disease Epidemiology," last modified October 15, 2012, http://www.epi.umn.edu/cvdepi/history-overview/.

48. A. Keys, C. Aravanis, H. W. Blackburn, F. S. Van Buchem, R. Buzina, B. D. Djordjević, A. S. Dontas, F. Fidanza, M. J. Karvonen, N. Kimura, D. Lekos, M. Monti, V. Puddu, and H. L. Taylor, "Epidemiological Studies Related to Coronary Heart Disease: Characteristics of Men Aged 40–59 in Seven Countries," *Acta Med Scand Suppl* 460 (1966): 1–392, https://doi.org/10.1111/j.0954-6820.1966.tb04737.x.

49. S. Ledermann, *Alcool, alcoolisme, alcoolisation*. (Paris: INED, 1956).

50. G. Rose and S. Day, "The Population Mean Predicts the Number of Deviant Individuals," *BMJ* 301(6759) (1990): 1031–1034, https://doi.org/10.1136/bmj.301.6759.1031.

51. G. Rose, *Rose's Strategy of Preventive Medicine* (Oxford: Oxford University Press, 2008), 102–103.

52. *Rose's Strategy of Preventive Medicine*, 142. See also M. G. Marmot, P. Elliott, M. J. Shipley, A. R. Dyer, H. Ueshima, D. G. Beevers, R. Stamler, H. Kesteloot, G. Rose, and J. Stamler, "Alcohol and Blood Pressure: The INTERSALT Study," *BMJ* 308(6939) (1994): 1263–1267, https://doi.org/10.1136/bmj.308.6939.1263.

53. *Rose's Strategy of Preventive Medicine*, 59.

54. G. Rose, "Strategy of Prevention: Lessons from Cardiovascular Disease," *BMJ* 282(6279) (1981): 1847–1851, https://doi.org/10.1136/bmj.282.6279.1847.

55. *Rose's Strategy of Preventive Medicine*, 129–140.

56. G. A. Mensah, G. S. Wei, P. D. Sorlie, L. J. Fine, Y. Rosenberg, P. G. Kaufmann, M. E. Mussolino, L. L. Hsu, E. Addou, M. M. Engelgau, and D. Gordon, "Decline in Cardiovascular Mortality: Possible Causes and Implications," *Circ Res* 120(2) (2017): 366–380, https://doi.org/10.1161/CIRCRESAHA.116.309115.

Chapter 7. HIV/AIDS

1. M. D. Grmek, *History of AIDS: Emergence and Origin of a Modern Pandemic* (Princeton, NJ: Princeton University Press, 1990).

2. J. Jones, C. Kelley, P. S. Sullivan, and J. W. Curran, "The Epidemiology and Prevention of HIV and AIDS," in *Maxcy-Rosenau-Last Public Health & Preventive Medicine*, 16th ed., ed. M. L. Boulton and R. B. Wallace, chap. 87 (New York: McGraw Hill, 2022).

3. Centers for Disease Control and Prevention, "Current Trends: Update on Acquired Immune Deficiency Syndrome (AIDS)—United States," *MMWR Weekly*, September 24, 1982, https://www.cdc.gov/mmwr/preview/mmwrhtml/00001163.htm.

4. O. Miettinen, "Estimability and Estimation in Case-Referent Studies," *Am. J Epidemiol* 103(2) (1976): 226–235, https://doi.org/10.1093/oxfordjournals.aje.a112220.

5. Grmek, *History of AIDS*; M. Marmor, A. E. Friedman-Kien, L. Laubenstein, R. D. Byrum, D. C. William, S. D'Onofrio, and N. Dubin, "Risk Factors for Kaposi's Sarcoma in Homosexual Men," *The Lancet* 319(8281) (1982): 1083–1087, https://doi.org/10.1016/s0140-6736(82)92275-9.

6. F. Barré-Sinoussi, J. C. Chermann, F. Rey, M. T. Nugeyre, S. Chamaret, J. Gruest, C. Dauguet, C. Axler-Blin, F. Vézinet-Brun, C. Rouzioux, W. Rozenbaum, and L. Montagnier, et al., "Isolation of a T-Lymphotropic Retrovirus from a Patient at Risk for Acquired Immune Deficiency Syndrome (AIDS)," *Science* 220(4599) (1983): 868–871, https://doi.org/10.1126/science.6189183.

7. B. D. Roberts, "HIV Antibody Testing Methods, 1985–1988," *J Insur Med* 26(1) (1994): 13–14.

8. L. B. Signorello, J. K. McLaughlin, L. Lipworth, S. Friis, H. T. Sørensen, and W. J. Blot, "Confounding by Indication in Epidemiologic Studies of Commonly Used Analgesics," *Am J Ther*, 2002. 9(3) (2002): 199–205, https://doi.org/10.1097/00045391-200205000 -00005.

9. J. B. Copas, "Randomization Models for the Matched and Unmatched 2 × 2 Tables," *Biometrika* 60 (1973): 467–476; D. B. Rubin, "Estimating Causal Effects of Treatments in Randomized and Nonrandomized Treatments," *J Educ Psychol* 66(5) (1974): 688–701; J. Splawa-Neyman, "On the Application of Probability Theory to Agricultural Experiments. Essay on Principles, Section 9," *Stat. Sci* 5(4) (1990): 465–480, https://doi.org/10.1214/ss/1177012032.

10. M. A. Hernán, "The C-Word: Scientific Euphemisms Do Not Improve Causal Inference from Observational Data," *Am J Public Health* 108(5) (2018): 616–619, https://doi.org/10.2105/AJPH .2018.304337.

11. J. Robins, "A New Approach to Causal Inference in Mortality Studies with Sustained Exposure Periods—Application to Control of the Healthy Worker Survivor Effect," *Math Model* 7(9–12) (1986): 1393–1512, https://doi.org/10.1016/0270-0255(86)90088-6.

12. Robins, "A New Approach to Causal Inference in Mortality Studies," 1436.

13. Robins, "A New Approach to Causal Inference in Mortality Studies," 1396.

14. The methods cannot be explained in a couple of paragraphs. Miguel Hernán and James Robins wrote a very clear and simple primer (M. A. Hernán and J. M. Robins, "Estimating Causal Effects from Epidemiological Data," *J. Epidemiol. Community Health* 60[7] [2006]: 578–586, https://doi.org/10.1136/jech.2004.029496). A textbook is in preparation (M. Hernán and J. M. Robins, *Causal Inference: What If?* [Boca Raton, FL, Chapman & Hall/CRC: in press]).

15. A. Park, "The Story Behind the First AIDS Drug," *Time*, March 19, 2017, https://time.com/4705809/first-aids-drug-azt/.

16. "Concorde: MRC/ANRS Randomised Double-Blind Controlled Trial of Immediate and Deferred Zidovudine in Symptom-Free HIV

Infection. Concorde Coordinating Committee," *The Lancet* 343(8902) (1994): 871–881, https://doi.org/10.1016/S0140 -6736(94)90006-X.

17. J. Robins, "The Analysis of Randomized and Nonrandomized AIDS Treatment Trials Using a New Approach to Causal Inference in Longitudinal Studies," in *Health Service Research Methodology: A Focus on AIDS*, ed. L. Sechrest, H. Freeman, and A. Mulley, 113–159 (Washington, DC: US Public Health Service, National Center for Health Services Research, 1989).

18. M. A. Hernáan, A. Alonso, R. Logan, F. Grodstein, K. B. Michels, W. C. Willett, J. E. Manson, and J. M. Robins, et al., "Observational Studies Analyzed Like Randomized Experiments: An Application to Postmenopausal Hormone Therapy and Coronary Heart Disease," *Epidemiology* 19(6) (2008): 766–779, https://doi.org/10.1097/EDE .0b013e3181875e61.

19. Hernáan and Robins, *Causal Inference: What If?* [in press].

Chapter 8. Social Determinants of Health

1. M. Marmot, *The Status Syndrome: How Social Standing Affects Our Health and Longevity* (New York: Henry Holt, 2004).

2. S. Galea and R. D. Vaughan, "Making the Invisible Causes of Population Health Visible: A Public Health of Consequence," *Am J Public Health* 108(8) (August 2018): 985–986.

3. US Department of Health and Human Services, Office of Disease Prevention and Health Promotion, "Healthy People 2030: Social Determinants of Health," https://health.gov/healthypeople/priority -areas/social-determinants-health.

4. A. Derickson, "'A Widespread Superstition': The Purported Invul- nerability of Workers of Color to Occupational Heat Stress," *Am J Public Health* 109(10) (2019): 1329–1335.

5. Derickson, "'A Widespread Superstition.'"

6. B. Hoffman, "Health Care Reform and Social Movements in the United States," *Am J Public Health* 93(1) (2003): 75–85.

7. A. Nelson, "The Longue Durée of Black Lives Matter," *Am J Public Health* 106(10) (2016): 1734–1737.

8. *Fatal Encounters*, https://fatalencounters.org/, accessed February 3, 2023.

9. *Mapping Police Violence*, "About This Project" (updated November 30, 2022), https://mappingpoliceviolence.org/about.

10. The 2020 Census counted a US population of 41,044,000 Black, 191,318,000 white, and 61,897,000 Hispanic people. For example, when the 500 killed white people are divided by the 191 million persons who identified as white in the 2020 Census, the killing yearly rate per million is 2.6 for whites. The corresponding annual rates are 6.7 for Blacks and 3.2 for Hispanics.

11.

Killed by police

YEAR	N			RATES / Million / year		
	BLACKS	WHITES	HISP	BLACKS	WHITES	HISP
2013	291	430	169	7.1	2.2	2.7
2014	276	480	183	6.7	2.5	3.0
2015	305	543	195	7.4	2.8	3.2
2016	279	533	195	6.8	2.8	3.2
2017	278	509	226	6.8	2.7	3.7
2018	265	512	213	6.5	2.7	3.4
2019	282	449	206	6.9	2.3	3.3
2020	249	412	201	6.1	2.2	3.2
2021	266	479	187	6.5	2.5	3.0
Total	**2,491**	**4,347**	**1,775**	**6.8**	**2.5**	**3.2**

Source: https://mappingpoliceviolence.org/

12. Mapping Police Violence, updated April 30, 2022, https://mappingpoliceviolence.org/.

13. Global Burden of Diseases 2019 Police Violence US Subnational Collaborators, "Fatal Police Violence by Race and State in the USA, 1980–2019: A Network Meta-Regression," *The Lancet*, 398(10307) (2021): 1239–1255; L. Peeples, "What the Data Say about Police Brutality and Racial Bias—and Which Reforms Might Work," *Nature* 583(7814) (2020): 22–24.

14. Federal Bureau of Prisons, "Statistics," last updated August 18, 2022, https://www.bop.gov/about/statistics/.

15. W. Sawyer and P. Wagner, "Mass Incarcerations: The Whole Pie, 2022," *Prison Policy Initiative*, March 14, 2022, https://www.prisonpolicy.org/reports/pie2022.html.

16. L. Brinkley-Rubinstein and D. H. Cloud, "Mass Incarceration as a Social-Structural Driver of Health Inequities: A Supplement to AJPH," *Am J Public Health* 110(S1) (2020): S14–S15.

17. K. Connors, M. H. Flores-Torres, D. Stern, U. Valdimarsdóttir, J. R. Rider, R. Lopez-Ridaura, C. Kirschbaum, C. Cantú-Brito, A. Catzin-Kuhlmann, B. L. Rodriguez, C. Pérez Correa, and M. Lajous, "Family Member Incarceration, Psychological Stress, and Subclinical Cardiovascular Disease in Mexican Women (2012–2016)," *Am J Public Health* 110(S1) (2020): S71–S77.

18. A. Case, and A. Deaton, "Rising Morbidity and Mortality in Midlife among White Non-Hispanic Americans in the 21st Century," *PNAS* 112(49) (2015): 15078–15083.

19. E. M. Stein, K. P. Gennuso, D. C. Ugboaja, and P. L. Remington, "The Epidemic of Despair among White Americans: Trends in the Leading Causes of Premature Death, 1999–2015," *Am J Public Health* 107(10) (2017): 1541–1547.

20. A. Case and A. Deaton, *Deaths of Despair and the Future of Capitalism* (Princeton, NJ: Princeton University Press, 2020).

21. Case and Deaton. *Deaths of Despair.*

22. Case and Deaton. *Deaths of Despair,* 172.

23. Jay Bhattacharya, Christina Gathmann, and Grant Miller, "The Gorbachev Anti-Alcohol Campaign and Russia's Mortality Crisis," *Am Econ J: Appl Econ* 5(2) (2013): 232–260, http://dx.doi.org/10.1257/app.5.2.232.

24. E. M. Stein, K. P. Gennuso, D. C. Ugboaja, and P. L. Remington, "The Epidemic of Despair among White Americans: Trends in the Leading Causes of Premature Death, 1999–2015," *Am J Public Health,* 107(10) (2017): 1541–1547. See also A. V. Diez Roux, "Despair as a Cause of Death: More Complex than It First Appears," *Am J Public Health* 107(10) (2017): 1566–1567.

25. S. Alang, T. B. Rogers, L. D. Williamson, C. Green, and A. J. Bell, "Police Brutality and Unmet Need for Mental Health Care," *Health Serv Res* 56(6): (2021): 1104–1113.

26. Johns Hopkins School of Public Health, Center for the Prevention of Youth Violence, "Safe Streets," https://www.jhsph.edu/research /centers-and-institutes/center-for-prevention-of-youth-violence /field_reports/Safe_Streets.html, accessed February 3, 2023.

27. L. Shanahan, S. N. Hill, L. M. Gaydosh, A. Steinhoff, E. J. Costello, K. A. Dodge, K. Mullan Harris, and W. E. Copeland, "Does Despair Really Kill? A Roadmap for an Evidence-Based Answer," *Am J Public Health* 109(6) (2019): 854–858.

28. J. W. Trotter, Jr., *Workers on Arrival: Black Labor in the Making of America* (Oakland: University of California Press, 2019).

29. E. M. Stein, K. P. Gennuso, D. C. Ugboaja, and P. L. Remington, "The Epidemic of Despair among White Americans: Trends in the Leading Causes of Premature Death, 1999–2015," *Am J Public Health* 107(10) (2017): 1541–1547.

30. R. Chetty, M. Stepner, S. Abraham, S. Lin, B. Scuderi, N. Turner, A. Bergeron, and D. Cutler, "The Association between Income and Life Expectancy in the United States, 2001–2014," *JAMA* 315(16) (2016): 1750–1766.

31. L. Gaydosh, R. A. Hummer, T. W. Hargrove, C. T. Halpern, J. M. Hussey, E. A. Whitsel, N. Dole, and K. Mullan Harris, "The Depths of Despair among US Adults Entering Midlife," *Am J Public Health* 109(5) (2019): 774–780.

32. S. H. Woolf, D. A. Chapman, J. M. Buchanich, K. J. Bobby, E. B Zimmerman, and S. M Blackburn, "Changes in Midlife Death Rates across Racial and Ethnic Groups in the United States: Systematic Analysis of Vital Statistics," *BMJ* 362 (2018): k3096.

33. Shanahan et al., "Does Despair Really Kill?"

34. Case and Deaton, *Deaths of Despair*.

Chapter 9. 1918 Influenza and SARS/COVID-19

1. World Health Organization, "The True Death Toll of COVID-19: Estimating Excess Mortality [in 2020]," https://www.who.int/data

/stories/the-true-death-toll-of-covid-19-estimating-global-excess
-mortality; United States Census Bureau, "Census Bureau Proj-
ects U.S. and World Populations on New Year's Day," December 30,
2019, https://www.census.gov/newsroom/press-releases/2019/new
-years-2020.html.

2. A picture of the industrial-scale, prolonged extreme overcrowding on
   US troopships is shown in C. A. Aligne, "Lost Lessons of the 1918
   Influenza: The 1920s Working Hypothesis, the Public Health Paradigm,
   and the Prevention of Deadly Pandemics," *Am J Public Health* 112(10)
   (2022): 1454–1464, https://doi.org/10.2105/AJPH.2022.306976.

3. A. Morabia, "The US Public Health Service House-to-House Canvass
   Survey of the Morbidity and Mortality of the 1918 Influenza Pandemic," *Am J Public Health* 111(3) (2021): 438–445, https://doi.org
   /10.2105/AJPH.2020.306025.

4. R. Pastor-Barriuso, B. Pérez-Gómez MD, J. Oteo-Iglesias,
   M. A. Hernán, M. Pérez-Olmeda, N. Fernández-de-Larrea,
   M. Molina, A. Fernández-García, M. Martín MEng, I. Cruz et al
   on behalf of the ENE-COVID Study Group. "Design and Implemen-
   tation of a Nationwide Population-Based Longitudinal Survey
   of SARS-CoV-2 Infection in Spain: The ENE-COVID Study", *Am
   J Public Health* 113 (5)(2023): 525-532, https://doi.org/10.2105
   /AJPH.2022.307167

5. Morabia, "The US Public Health Service House-to-House Canvass
   Survey," 444.

6. R. Fisher, "The Fiasco of the 1976 'Swine Flu Affair,'" *BBC News,*
   September 21, 2020, https://www.bbc.com/future/article/20200918
   -the-fiasco-of-the-us-swine-flu-affair-of-1976.

7. J. Sturcke, "Bird Flu Pandemic 'Could Kill 150m,'" *The Guardian,*
   September 30, 2005, https://www.theguardian.com/world/2005
   /sep/30/birdflu.jamessturcke; T. Jefferson, M. Jones, P. Doshi and
   C. Del Mar, "Neuraminidase Inhibitors for Preventing and Treating
   Influenza in Healthy Adults: Systematic Review and Meta-Analysis,"
   BMJ 339 (2009): b5106, https://doi.org/10.1136/bmj.b5106.

8. M. Greenberger, "Better Prepare than React: Reordering Public
   Health Priorities 100 Years after the Spanish Flu Epidemic," *Am J*

Public Health 108(11) (2018): 1465–1468 (1467), https://doi.org /10.2105/AJPH.2018.304682.

9. B. J. Jester, T. M. Uyeki, A. Patel, L. Koonin, and D. B. Jernigan, "100 Years of Medical Countermeasures and Pandemic Influenza Preparedness," *Am J Public Health* 108(11) (2018): 1469–1472, https://doi.org/10.2105/AJPH.2018.304586.

10. J. L. Schwartz, "The Spanish Flu, Epidemics, and the Turn to Biomedical Responses," *Am J Public Health* 108(11) (2018): 1455– 1458, https://doi.org/10.2105/AJPH.2018.304581.

11. W. E. Parmet, and M. A. Rothstein, "The 1918 Influenza Pandemic: Lessons Learned and Not—Introduction to the Special Section," *Am J Public Health* 108(11) (2018): 1435–1436, https://doi.org/10 .2105/AJPH.2018.304695. See also D. M. Lazer, J., M. A. Baum, Y. Benkler, A. J. Berinsky, K. M. Greenhill, F. Menczer, M. J. Metzger, B. Nyhan, G. Pennycook, D. Rothschild, et al., "The Science of Fake News," *Science* 359(6380) (2018): 1094–1096, https://doi.org /10.1126/science.aao2998D; A. Broniatowski, A. M. Jamison, S. Qi, L. AlKulaib, T. Chen, A. Benton, S. C. Quinn, and M. Dredze, "Weaponized Health Communication: Twitter Bots and Russian Trolls Amplify the Vaccine Debate," *Am J Public Health* 108(10) (2018): 1378–1384, https://doi.org/10.2105/AJPH.2018.304567.

12. D. U. Himmelstein, and S. Woolhandler, "Public Health's Falling Share of US Health Spending," *Am J Public Health* 106(1) (2016): 56–57, https://doi.org/10.2105/AJPH.2015.302908.

13. G. Wilensky, "The Importance of Reestablishing a Pandemic Prepared- ness Office at the White House," *JAMA Health Forum* 1(7) (2020): e200864, https://doi.org/10.1001/jamahealthforum.2020.0864.

14. Statista Research Department, "Number of People without Health Insurance in the United States from 1997 to 2021," August 29, 2022, https://www.statista.com/statistics/200955/americans-without -health-insurance/.

15. K. E. W. Himmelstein and A. S. Venkataramani, "Economic Vulner- ability among US Female Health Care Workers: Potential Impact of a $15-per-Hour Minimum Wage," *Am J Public Health* 109(2) (2019): 198–205, https://doi.org/10.2105/AJPH.2018.304801.

16. M. A. Rothstein and C. N. Coughlin, "Ensuring Compliance with Quarantine by Undocumented Immigrants and Other Vulnerable Groups: Public Health Versus Politics," *Am J Public Health* 109(9) (2019): 1179–1183. Articles in the December 2022 issue of the *American Journal of Public Health* show some of the harmful effects of the threat: D. P. Miller, R. S. John, M. Yao, and M. Morris, "The 2016 Presidential Election, the Public Charge Rule, and Food and Nutrition Assistance among Immigrant Households," *Am J Public Health* 112(12) (2022):1738–1746, https://doi.org/10.2105/AJPH.2022.307011; S. S. Wang, S. Glied, C. Babcock, and A. Chaudry, "Changes in the Public Charge Rule and Health of Mothers and Infants Enrolled in New York State's Medicaid Program, 2014–2019," *Am J Public Health* 112(12) (2022): 1747–1756, https://doi.org/10.2105/AJPH.2022.307066; E. DeGarmo, J. Rosen, and L. Rutkow, "Use of Law by US States during the COVID-19 Pandemic with Respect to People Who Were Undocumented," *Am J Public Health* 112(12) (2022):1757–1764, https://doi.org /10.2105/AJPH.2022.307090.

17. M. A. Rothstein and C. N. Coughlin, "Ensuring Compliance with Quarantine by Undocumented Immigrants and Other Vulnerable Groups: Public Health versus Politics," *Am J Public Health* 109(9) (2019): 1179–1183 (1180), https://doi.org/10.2105/AJPH.2019.305201

18. "How Epidemiology Has Shaped the COVID Pandemic," *Nature* 589(7843) (2021): 491–492, https://doi.org/10.1038/d41586-021 -00183-z.

19. J. T. Wu, K. Leung, and G. M. Leung, "Nowcasting and Forecasting the Potential Domestic and International Spread of the 2019-nCoV Outbreak Originating in Wuhan, China: A Modelling Study," *The Lancet* 395(10225) (2020): 689–697, https://doi.org/016/S0140 -6736(20)30260-9.

20. See, for example, S. Richardson, J. S. Hirsch, M. Narasimhan, J. M. Crawford, T. McGinn, K. W. Davidson, and the Northwell COVID-19 Research Consortium, "Presenting Characteristics, Comorbidities, and Outcomes among 5700 Patients Hospitalized with COVID-19 in the New York City Area," *JAMA* 323(20) (2020): 2052–2059, https://doi.org/10.1001/jama.2020.6775.

21. E. Banco, "Inside America's Covid-Reporting Breakdown," *Politico*, August 15, 2021, https://www.politico.com/news/2021/08/15/inside -americas-covid-data-gap-502565.

22. S. Toy, "CDC Director Aims to Improve Covid-19 Messaging, Data Collection," *Wall Street Journal*, January 17, 2022, https://www.wsj .com/articles/cdc-director-aims-to-improve-covid-19-messaging -data-collection-11642429801.

23. N. Pearce, J. P. Vandenbroucke, T. J. VanderWeele, and S. Greenland, "Accurate Statistics on COVID-19 Are Essential for Policy Guidance and Decisions," *Am J Public Health* 110(7) (2020): 949–951, https://doi.org/10.2105/AJPH.2020.305708.

24. Pearce et al., "Accurate Statistics on COVID-19 Are Essential."

25. L. Bowleg, "We're Not All in This Together: On COVID-19, Intersectionality, and Structural Inequality," *Am J Public Health* 110(7) (2020): 917, https://doi.org/10.2105/AJPH.2020.305766.

26. N. Krieger, "ENOUGH: COVID-19, Structural Racism, Police Brutality, Plutocracy, Climate Change-and Time for Health Justice, Democratic Governance, and an Equitable, Sustainable Future. *Am J Public Health* 110(11) (2020): 1620–1623, https://doi.org/10.2105 /AJPH.2020.305886.

27. D. T. Lau, P. Sosa, N. Dasgupta, and H. He, "Impact of the CO-VID-19 Pandemic on Public Health Surveillance and Survey Data Collections in the United States," *Am J Public Health* 111(12) (2021): 2118–2121, https://doi.org/10.2105/AJPH.2021.306551.

28. P. Elliott, M. Whitaker, D. Tang, O. Eales, N. Steyn, B. Bodinier, H. Wang, J. Elliott, C. Atchison, D. Ashby, et al., "Design and Implementation of a National SARS-CoV-2 Monitoring Program in England: REACT-1 Study", *Am J Public Health* 113 (5) (2023): 545-554, https://doi.org/10.2105/AJPH.2023.307230. K. B. Pouwels, T. House, E. Pritchard, et al., "Community Prevalence of SARS-CoV-2 in England from April to November 2020: Results from the ONS Coronavirus Infection Survey," *Lancet Public Health* 6 (1) (2021): e30–e8, https://doi.org/10.1016/S2468-2667(20)30282-6. See also the argument in favor of random sampling: N. Dean, "Tracking COVID-19 Infections: Time for Change," *Nature*

602(7896) (2022): 185, https://doi.org/10.1038/d41586-022
-00336-8.

29. Estudio Nacional de sero-Epidemiología de la Infección por
SARS-CoV-2 en España (ENE-Covid), https://www.sanidad.gob.es
/ciudadanos/ene-covid/home.htm. See M. Pollán, B. Pérez-Gómez,
R. Pastor-Barriuso, J. Oteo, M. A. Hernán, M. Pérez-Olmeda, J. L.
Sanmartín, A. Fernández-García, I. Cruz, N. Fernández de Larrea,
et al., "Prevalence of SARS-CoV-2 in Spain (ENE-COVID): A
Nationwide, Population-Based Seroepidemiological Study," *The
Lancet* 396(10250) (2020): 535–544, https://doi.org/10.1016
/S0140-6736(20)31483-5.

30. For more about the CDC's plan for accomplishing this goal, see
Centers for Disease Control and Prevention, "Data Modernization
Initiative," last reviewed May 10, 2022, https://www.cdc.gov
/surveillance/data-modernization/index.html; and Centers for
Disease Control and Prevention, "DMI Modernization Snapshot,"
last reviewed March 30, 2022, https://www.cdc.gov/surveillance
/pubs-resources/dmi_snapshot.html.

Epilogue

1. A. Remmel, "Why Is It So Hard to Investigate the Rare Side Effects
of COVID Vaccines?" *Nature*, April 1, 2021, https://doi.org/10.1038
/d41586-021-00880-9.

2. M. Astor, "Vaccination Mandates Are an American Tradition; So Is the
Backlash," *New York Times*. September 9, 2021, https://www.nytimes
.com/2021/09/09/us/politics/vaccine-mandates-history.html.

3. Jacobsen v. Massachusetts, 197 U.S. 11 (1905), https://supreme.justia
.com/cases/federal/us/197/11/.

4. J. Colgrove and R. Bayer, "Manifold Restraints: Liberty, Public
Health, and the Legacy of *Jacobson v Massachusetts*." *Am J Public
Health* 95(4) (2005): 571–576, https://doi.org/10.2105/AJPH.2004
.055145.

5. L. O. Gostin, "*Jacobson v Massachusetts* at 100 Years: Police Power
and Civil Liberties in Tension," *Am J Public Health* 95(4) (2005):
576–581, https://doi.org/10.2105/AJPH.2004.055152.

6. W. K. Mariner, G. J. Annas, and L. H. Glantz, "*Jacobson v Massachusetts:* It's Not Your Great-Great-Grandfather's Public Health Law," *Am J Public Health* 95(4) (2005): 581–590, https://doi.org/10.2105 /AJPH.2004.055160.

7. Colgrove and Bayer, "Manifold Restraints."

8. J. H. Jones, *Bad Blood: The Tuskegee Syphilis Experiment*, new and expanded edition (New York: Free Press, 1993).

9. V. N. Gamble, "Under the Shadow of Tuskegee: African Americans and Health Care," *Am J Public Health*," 87(11) (1997): 1773–1778.

10. M. A. Rodriguez, and R. García, "First, Do No Harm: The US Sexually Transmitted Disease Experiments in Guatemala," *Am J Public Health* 103(12) (2013): 2122–2126, https://doi.org/10.2105 /AJPH.2013.301520.

11. N. L. Novak, N. Lira, K. E. O'Connor, S. D. Harlow, S. L. R. Kardia, and A. M. Stern, "Disproportionate Sterilization of Latinos under California's Eugenic Sterilization Program, 1920–1945," *Am J Public Health* 108(5) (2018): 611–613, https://doi.org/10.2105/AJPH .2018.304369; A. M. Stern, "Sterilized in the Name of Public Health: Race, Immigration, and Reproductive Control in Modern California," *Am J Public Health* 95(7) (2005): 1128–1138, https://doi.org /10.2105/AJPH.2004.041608; A. M. Stern, N. L. Novak, N. Lira, K. O'Connor, S. Harlow, and S. Kardia, "California's Sterilization Survivors: An Estimate and Call for Redress," *Am J Public Health* 107(1) (2017): 50–54, https://doi.org/10.2105/AJPH.2016.303489.

12. E. K. Abel, "'Only the best class of immigration': Public Health Policy toward Mexicans and Filipinos in Los Angeles, 1910–1940," *Am J Public Health* 94(6) (2004): 932–939, https://doi.org/10.2105 /ajph.94.6.932.

13. S. M. Reverby, "Historical Misfeasance: Immorality to Justice in Public Health," *Am J Public Health* 107(1) (2017): 14–15 (15), https://doi.org/10.2105/AJPH.2016.303554. See also S. M. Reverby, "Ethical Failures and History Lessons: The US Public Health Service Research Studies in Tuskegee and Guatemala," *Public Health Reviews* 34(1) (2012): 1–18, https://doi.org/10.1007/BF03391665.

14. K. W. Crenshaw, "Mapping the Margins: Intersectionality, Identity Politics, and Violence against Women of Color," *Stanford Law Rev.* 43(6) (1991): 1241–1299, https://doi.org/10.2307 /1229039.

15. L. Bowleg, "The Problem with the Phrase *Women and Minorities*: Intersectionality—An Important Theoretical Framework for Public Health," *Am J Public Health*, 102(7) (2012): 1267–1273, https://doi .org/10.2105/AJPH.2012.300750

16. R. Bayer, "Public Health Policy and the AIDS Epidemic: An End to HIV Exceptionalism?" *N Engl J Med* 324(21) (1991): 1500–1504, https://doi.org/10.1056/NEJM199105233242111.

17. S. Epstein, *Impure Science: AIDS, Activism, and the Politics of Knowledge* (Berkeley: University of California Press, 1998).

18. D. D. Diallo, "The Sankofa Paradox: Why Black Women Know the HIV Epidemic Ends with 'WE.' *Am J Public Health* 111(7) (2021): 1237–1239, https://doi.org/10.2105/AJPH.2021.306358.

19. C. Levenstein, L. I. Boden, and D. H. Wegman, "COSH: A Grass- Roots Public Health Movement," *Am J Public Health* 74(9) (1984): 964–965, https://doi.org/10.2105/ajph.74.9.964.

20. M. Kiser and K. Lovelace, "A National Network of Public Health and Faith-Based Organizations to Increase Influenza Prevention among Hard-to-Reach Populations," *Am J Public Health* 109(3) (2019): 371–377, https://doi.org/10.2105/AJPH.2018.304826.

21. S. Landers and F. Kapadia, "50 Years after Stonewall, the LGBTQ Health Movement Embodies Empowerment, Expertise, and Energy," *Am J Public Health* 109(6) (2019): 849–850, https://doi.org /10.2105/AJPH.2019.305087.

22. A. J. Martos, P. A. Wilson, and I. H. Meyer, "Lesbian, Gay, Bisexual, and Transgender (LGBT) Health Services in the United States: Origins, Evolution, and Contemporary Landscape," *PLOS One* 12(7) (2017), https://doi.org10.1371/journal.pone.0180544.

23. P. N. Halkitis, "The Stonewall Riots, the AIDS Epidemic, and the Public's Health," *Am J Public Health* 109(6) (2019): 851–852, https://doi.org/10.2105/AJPH.2019.305079.

24. Diallo, "The Sankofa Paradox," 1238. Diallo is the founder and president of SisterLove, an organization that focuses on the needs of women living with AIDS.

25. Levenstein, Boden, and Wegman, "COSH: A Grass-Roots Public Health Movement," 965.

26. Kiser and Lovelace. "A National Network of Public Health and Faith-Based Organizations."

27. C. A. Roberto and J. L. Pomeranz, "Public Health and Legal Arguments in Favor of a Policy to Cap the Portion Sizes of Sugar-Sweetened Beverages," *Am J Public Health* 105(11) (2015): 2183–2190, https://doi.org/10.2105/AJPH.2015.302862.

28. M. Nestle, *Soda Politics: Taking on Big Soda (and Winning)* (New York: Oxford University Press, 2015).

29. Nestle, *Soda Politics,* 359.

30. K. Sellers, J. P. Leider, E. Gould, B. C. Castrucci, A. Beck, K. Bogaert, F. Coronado, G. Shah, V. Yeager, L. M. Beitsch, and P. C. Erwin, "The State of the US Governmental Public Health Workforce, 2014–2017," *Am J Public Health* 109(5) (2019): 674–680, https://doi.org/10.2105/AJPH.2019.305011.

31. J. A. Ward, E. M. Stone, P. Mui, and B. Resnick, "Pandemic-Related Workplace Violence and Its Impact on Public Health Officials, March 2020–January 2021," *Am J Public Health* 112 (2022): 736–746, https://doi.org/10.2105/AJPH.2021.306649.

32. The quote is on minute 6′ 26″ of the Youtube podcast, American Journal of Public Health, "Harassment of Public Health Officials," https://www.youtube.com/watch?v=1gPxhTz8iIU. The transcript is available at https://ajph.aphapublications.org/pb-assets/podcasts/2022/Transcripts/AJPH_July2022_Podcast_Harassment_Transcript-1663215034.pdf.

33. P. C. Erwin, A. J. Beck, V. A. Yeager, and J. P. Leider, "Public Health Undergraduates in the Workforce: A Trickle, Soon a Wave?" *Am J Public Health* 109(5) (2019): 685–687, https://doi.org/10.2105/AJPH.2019.305004; B. Resnick, J. P. Leider, and R. Riegelman, "The Landscape of US Undergraduate Public Health Education,"

Public Health Rep 133(5) (2018): 619–628, https://doi.org
/10.1177/0033354918784911.

34. Council on Education for Public Health, "List of Accredited Schools and Programs," https://ceph.org/about/org-info/who-we-accredit /accredited/.

35. See Institute of Medicine, Committee for the Study of the Future of Public Health, *The Future of Public Health* (Washington, DC: National Academies Press, 1988); Institute of Medicine, *For the Public's Health: Investing in a Healthier Future* (Washington, DC: National Academies Press, 2012).

36. S. Magnan and S. M. Teutsch, "Changing the Public's Health Story: Reducing Wasteful Medical Care Spending—Introduction to the Special *AJPH* Section," *Am J Public Health* 110(12) (2020): 1731–1732, https://doi.org/10.2105/AJPH.2020.305984; M. Speer, J. M. McCullough, J. E. Fielding, E. Faustino, and S. M Teutsch, "Excess Medical Care Spending: The Categories, Magnitude, and Opportunity Costs of Wasteful Spending in the United States," *Am J Public Health* 110(12) (2020): 1743–1748, https://doi.org/10.2105/AJPH .2020.305865.

37. R. C. Brownson, T. A. Burke, G. A. Colditz, and J. M. Samet, "Reimagining Public Health in the Aftermath of a Pandemic," *Am J Public Health* 110(11) (2020): 1605–1610, https://doi.org/10.2105 /AJPH.2020.305861.

Appendix. How Old Is the Public Health Approach?

1. G. Rosen, *A History of Public Health* (Baltimore, MD: Johns Hopkins University Press, 1993); D. Porter, *Health, Civilization, and the State: A History of Public Health from Ancient to Modern Times* (London: Routledge, 1999).

2. A. Morabia, *Enigmas of Health and Disease: How Epidemiology Helps Unravel Scientific Mysteries* (New York: Columbia University Press, 2014), 205–210.

3. W. H. McNeill, *Plagues and Peoples* (New York: Anchor Books, 1977).

4. McNeill, *Plagues and Peoples*.

5. McNeill, *Plagues and Peoples*, 78

6. McNeill, *Plagues and Peoples*, 259–269.

7. A. Morabia, "Epidemic and Population Patterns in the Chinese Empire (243 B.C.E. to 1911 C.E.): Quantitative Analysis of a Unique but Neglected Epidemic Catalogue," *Epidemiol Infect* 137(10) (2009): 1361–1368, https://doi.org/10.1017 /S0950268809990136.

8. A. Morabia, *Enigmas of Health and Disease: How Epidemiology Helps Unravel Scientific Mysteries* (New York: Columbia University Press, 2014).

9. My preferred translation of some Hippocratic Treatises exists only in French by Jacques Jouanna (https://www.lesbelleslettres.com /contributeur/jacques-jouanna). Translations of snippets from Jouanna exist in English, but not for all the texts I am citing in this chapter. I highly recommend J. Jouanna, *Hippocrates* (Medicine and Culture series) (Baltimore, MD: Johns Hopkins University Press, 1998). The systematic English translations, which I am referring to, are not reader friendly. The original doctors certainly did not speak like these translations make them sound. A fresh translation is warranted.

10. I. B. Cohen, *The Triumph of Numbers* (New York: Norton, 2005), 28–31. The story is recorded in two different ways in the Old Testament: in 2 Sam. 24:1–25 and in 1 Chron. 21:1–30.

11. M. A. Greenwood, "Statistical Mare's Nest?" *J R Stat Soc* 103(2) (1940): 246–248, https://doi.org/10.2307/2980417; P. Pflaumer, "Estimations of the Roman Life Expectancy Using Ulpian's Table," unpublished paper (2015), https://eldorado.tu-dortmund.de /bitstream/2003/34384/1/JSM2015Pflaumer.pdf.

12. Hippocrates, *Of the Epidemics*, book I, section 1, paragraph 1: First constitution, trans Frances Adams. http://classics.mit.edu /Hippocrates/epidemics.1.i.html.

13. H. E. Sigerist, *A History of Medicine*, 1: *Primitive and Archaic Medicine* (New York: Oxford University Press, 1951), 65.

14. Mumps became a childhood disease in large populations when most adults became immune to it. Thanks to the measles, mumps, and

rubella (MMR) vaccine, outbreaks of mumps have become rare. A. Hviid, S. Rubin, and K. Mühlemann, "Mumps," *The Lancet* 371(9616) (2008): 932–944, https://doi.org/10.1016/S0140 -6736(08)60419-5.

15. However, this is different from saying, as a modern assessment of the symptoms and signs of mumps would, that 60%–70% of mumps infections are symptomatic, that parotitis generally occurs in 95% of children with clinical symptoms, and that epididymo-orchitis occurs in 15%–30% of symptomatic cases and is bilateral in 15%–30% of those cases (that is, in 5%–10% of all symptomatic cases). These modern statistics may not be directly comparable to those that a Hippocratic doctor could have computed, since in 500 BCE, mumps was a universal disease, but it has become a childhood infection.

16. There exist multiple interpretations of the concept of miasma in Hippocrates' writing besides that it is a physical and natural cause. See J. Jouanna, "Air, Miasma and Contagion in the Time of Hippocrates and the Survival of Miasmas in Post-Hippocratic Medicine (Rufus of Ephesus, Galen and Palladius)," in *Greek Medicine from Hippocrates to Galen*, ed. J. Jouanna, 119–136 (Leiden: Brill, 2012), https://doi.org/10.1163/9789004232549_008.

17. Joanna, *Hippocrates*, 205.

18. Hippocrates, *Nature of Man*, vol. 4, Loeb Classical Library, no. 150 (Boston, MA: Harvard University Press, 1931), 25, https://archive.org /details/hippocrates04hippuoft/page/24/mode/2up?view=theater.

19. Hippocrates, *Nature of Man*, 4:25.

20. Hippocrates, *On Airs, Waters, Places*, trans. Frances Adams (London, 1881), http://classics.mit.edu/Hippocrates/airwatpl.html.

21. Hippocrates, *On Airs, Waters, Places*, part 24.

22. Hippocrates, *On Airs, Waters, Places*, part 16.

23. Hippocrates, *On Airs, Waters, Places*, part 16.

24. S. Weingarten, "Food in Daniel 1:1–16: The First Controlled Experiment?" *JLL Bulletin: Commentaries on the History of Treatment Evaluation* (2004) https://www.jameslindlibrary.org/articles/food -daniel-15-16-first-report-controlled-experiment/).

25. A. M. Lilienfeld, "The Fielding H. Garrison Lecture: *Ceteris paribus:* The Evolution of the Clinical Trial," *Bull Hist Med* 56(1) (1982): 1–18 (5).

26. P. E. Pormann, "Qualifying and Quantifying Medical Uncertainty in 10th Century Baghdad: Abu Bakr al-Razi," *J R Soc Med* 112(4) (2019): 160–163, https://doi.org/10.1177/0141076813496515.

27. Pormann, "Qualifying and Quantifying Medical Uncertainty," 160.

28. Quoted in I. M. Donaldson, "Petrarch's letter to Boccaccio 'On the Proud and Presumptuous Behaviour of Physicians,'" *J R Soc Med* 109(9) (2016): 347–353, https://doi.org/10.1177/0892705716663088.

29. C. Solís, "Bartolomé Hidalgo de Agüero's 16th Century, Evidence-Based Challenge to the Orthodox Management of Wounds," *J R Soc Med* 105(9) (2012): 401–402, https://doi.org/10.1258/jrsm.2012.12k062.

30. Bartolomé Hidalgo de Agüero, *Tesoro de la verdadera cirugía y vía particular contra la común* (Seville: Francisco Pérez, 1604), 32v.

31. Solís, "Bartolomé Hidalgo de Agüero," 402.

32. P. D. Mitchell, "Human Parasites in the Roman World: Health Consequences of Conquering an Empire," *Parasitology* 144(1) (2017): 48–58, https://doi.org/10.1017/S0031182015001651.

33. Mitchell, "Human Parasites in the Roman World," 48.

34. H. R. Harvey, "Public Health in Aztec Society," *Bull N Y Acad Med* 57(2) (1981): 157–165.

35. J. Snow, *On the Mode of Communication of Cholera*. 2nd ed. (London: Churchill, 1855). About the fact that the Lambeth filtered its water, see "Southwark and Vauxhall Water Company: Brief History [of the Lambeth Waterworks] during the Snow Era (1813–1858)," undated, https://www.ph.ucla.edu/epi/snow/1859map/lambeth_waterworks_a2.html (accessed February 5, 2023).

Index

Figures, notes, and tables are indicated by *f, n,* and *t* following the page number.